The Way to Good Health with Chinese Herbs

Hong-yen Hsu, Ph.D.

Oriental Healing Arts Institute

ABOUT THE AUTHOR

Dr. Hong-yen Hsu has a distinguished background in research and teaching. After graduation from the Meiji Pharmaceutical College and the Pharmacognosy Department of Tokyo University, Dr. Hsu earned his Doctor of Pharmacy degree at the University of Kyoto. He remained in Japan for three more years as a member of the research staff of the Department of Pharmaceutical Science at the University of Tokyo, before returning to Taiwan in 1945. Since that time he has been actively engaged in teaching and conducting research at National Taiwan University, and the Medical Colleges at Taipei, Taichung, and Kaohsiung. Dr. Hsu is Dean of the Botany Department at the College of Chinese Culture, Director of the Institute of Pharmacological Science at the China Medical College, and President of the Oriental Healing Arts Institute. A prolific author, he has published more than one hundred articles and books.

NOTICE

Information compiled from traditional medical texts and from the observations of modern authorities on Chinese medicine is presented here for its educational value and should not be used for treatment or prevention of disease without the advice of a Chinese physician or other medical authority.

ISBN: 0-941 942-01-5

CONTENTS

PREFACE

It is my earnest hope that the reader will find this a practical and easily understood reference to Chinese herbal medicine. I am particularly pleased to add diet therapy to the sparse material available in English on that subject. Nutrition remains an integral part of Chinese medicine: the philosophy of health as balance has been present in Chinese culture for centuries. Through extensive clinical experience, Chinese doctors long ago put into practice concepts just recently explored by Western scientists.

Originally published in Chinese, ***The Way to Good Health with Chinese Herbs*** *was translated into English by the staff of the Brion Research Institute in Taiwan and edited by Nancy Hays and Judith Haueter of the Oriental Healing Arts Institute in Los Angeles. The editors organized the English edition in alphabetical order for quick and easy reference. Let me note here that the first formula(s) listed under each disease name should be tried first and that one of the alternate formulas should be chosen only if the formula of choice proves ineffective.*

I believe that there is a great deal more that the West can learn from the East and will do my best to promote such an exchange of ideas.

— Hong-yen Hsu
December 1981

I. DIET AND HEALTH

Chinese medical theory contends that diseases are caused by environmental elements (wind, cold, moisture, heat, aridity, and fire) and by internal factors (pleasure, anger, anxiety, pensiveness, sorrow, fear, and terror). Treatment focuses not only on eliminating harmful toxins but also on strengthening vitality and the body's resistance to disease. Western treatment, on the other hand, mostly adopts palliative localized treatment, treating the head for headaches and the feet for aching feet. Chinese medicine seeks a whole body treatment, or a radical treatment, by adjusting the imbalance in the body that is causing the headache or the aching feet. Radical treatment employs not only medicines but also diet and exercise in therapy. *Su wen*, the fountainhead of Chinese medicine, propounds: "Attack harmful toxins with poisons (drugs); nourish the body with the five grains; assist the nourishment with the five animals and five fruits; enrich the effect with the five vegetables; supplement essence and *ch'i* by matching appropriately odors and tastes."

Some combinations of herbs designed for removing harmful toxins damage the body. Therefore, formulas should be prescribed in accordance with specific foods, taking into account taste and character so as to supplement and strengthen the sperm and *ch'i* and nourish the body.

Chinese physicians outlined basic therapy two thousand years ago in the *Su wen* and *Shen nung pen ts'ao ching*. The concepts are exclusive to Chinese medicine. The taste and smell of foods and herbal drugs correspond to the "four energies" and "five tastes." The four energies are cold, hot, warm, and cool while the five tastes are sour, bitter, pungent, salty, and sweet. Cool herbs and foods treat febrile diseases. Hot herbs and foods remedy cold diseases. Sweet food and drugs disperse, promote circulation, nourish the body, and harmonize the stomach. Bitter foods and drugs solidify and purge; harsh, sour drugs and food astringe and solidify; and salty ones soften and purge. Some herbs with a pungent smell, like fresh ginger, perilla, and mentha, are used to disperse external toxins. Sweet herbs are tonics and lenitives; for example, ginseng nourishes *ch'i* and licorice works as a paregoric. Bitter herbs, such as coptis and bittermelon, have drying and purging actions. Rhubarb regulates the bowels and purges firm fevers. The skin of pomegranate, sour and harsh, stops prolonged diarrhea and heals anal prolapse. Kelp is salty and softens, solidifies, and moistens. It is used to treat stagnant sputum and scrofula. Bland herbs, those with no taste such as hoelen and akebia, are diuretics.

Cool natured foods include pears, oranges, watermelon, bittermelon, long crooked squash, eggplant, green lentils, bean curd, and bamboo. Cabbage, leek, pumpkin, fresh ginger, vinegar, and pepper moisten. Mild, warm foods are chicken and beef, while hot foods include wine, mutton, and dog meat. Included in the sweet foods are corn, sweet potatoes, peas, jujube, dates, longan, and trapa. Olives are considered to be sour. Thus in order to maintain one's health, a person chooses suitable foods according to his individual physical condition.

Eating and drinking indiscriminantly injures the spleen and stomach and changes the metabolism, predisposing one to disease. For example, frequent consumption of fatty food causes wet fever, gastric injury, heartburn, congestion, and chest stagnancy which in turn cause carbuncles and abscesses. An excess of pungent food incites fever in the gastrointestinal tract, stomach upsets, and hemorrhoids. Too much sour food injures the spleen; too much bitter food, the liver; and too much salt, the heart. Heavy drinking of alcoholic beverages damages the *ch'i* and blood and causes wine gangrene and mental illness.

Labor is instinctive to human beings and plays an important role in life. The *Su wen* says: "Excessive leisure and ease cause circulatory problems and a subsequent loss of health. However, too much work exhausts the *ch'i* and blood and injures the sinews and bones." Moderation is the key to long life.

The lack of exercise, especially the lack of walking, predisposes a middle-aged person to heart disease and arteriosclerosis. Aging begins in the feet. Thus walking is the best exercise. In general the average person walks 3-6,000 steps a day. The ideal is 10,000 steps a day. Walking increases both breathing and pulse rates. On the average a person's pulse rate should be 70 at rest, 90-100 when walking, and 120-130 when jogging. After trotting, a person over sixty will have a rate of about 110. Of course, one should not exercise beyond his physical capacity. It is important to adjust the speed of one's walking with the pulse rate and to walk every day or at least every other day.

Thus the way to good health lies in harmonizing one's physical body with proper diet, work, and exercise.

II. DIET THERAPY FOR MAJOR DISEASES

HYPERTENSION, ARTERIOSCLEROSIS

Generally, a low salt, restricted calorie diet; reduced consumption of alcohol; low cholesterol, low-fat foods; vegetable rather than animal fat; lean meat; high vitamin content vegetables.

Allowable Foods:

Grains: cooked rice, bread, noodles
Vegetables: spinach, carrots, turnips, pumpkin, peas, tomatoes
Fruits: apples, oranges, grapes, pears, loquats, apricots, peaches, cumquats
Dairy products: regular or skim milk, goat's milk
Seaweed: kelp
Others: bean curd

Foods To Be Avoided:

Meats: beef, pork, liver, sausage, preserved meat, gravy
Animal fat, especially lard
Salt-preserved food
Beverages: wine, coffee, tea, carbonated drinks
Spices: pepper, mustard, capsicum, wasabia

Foods To Be Restricted:

White fish: dab, flounder
Eggs: chicken, duck
Vegetable oils: bean, sesame
Spices: salt, mayonnaise, spices in general
Sweets: syrup, cookies, sweets in general
Water: 1.5 liters a day

NEPHRITIS

Reduced salt, low-fat, high-protein diet.

Allowable Foods:

Grains: soft rice, rice gruel, noodles
Vegetables: cabbage, spinach, turnips, carrots, potatoes, sweet potatoes, dioscorea (Chinese potatoes and yams)
Fruits: apples, oranges, peaches, grapes
Others: bean curd, vinegar, sugar, fat

Foods To Be Avoided

Meats: fish, gravy
Salty food: salt, soy sauce, miso, salt-containing or salt-preserved food
Stimulants: wine, coffee, thick tea, mustard, pepper

DIABETES MELLITUS

Restricted sugar, low-calorie, low-carbohydrate (150-250 grams) diet; 1.5 grams of protein per kilogram body weight; most fruits allowed.

Allowable Foods:

Vegetables: onion, bamboo, spinach, cabbage, turnips, cucumber, eggplant, asparagus, other low carbohydrate vegetables
Beverages: wine, coffee, black tea

Foods To Be Avoided:

Vegetables: potatoes, sweet potatoes, arctium, lotus root, dioscorea, taro
Fruits: bananas, persimmons, grapes
Spices: salt, miso, pepper, cayenne pepper, mustard
Sweets: all

OBESITY

Low-calorie diet, reduced salt and liquids.

Allowable Foods:

Low-fat foods
Lean meat
Fish: shrimp, conch
Others: skim milk, bean curd, tea and coffee without sugar

Foods To Be Avoided:

High-fat and high-carbohydrate foods
Grains: overconsumption of rice
Vegetables: potatoes, sweet potatoes, beans
Fruits: grapes, peaches
Sweets: especially cocoa, chocolate, cookies
Beverages: wine

HEPATITIS, CIRRHOSIS

High-protein, high-calorie diet of light smelling foods; no smoking.

Allowable Foods:

Meats: chicken, liver
Vegetables: spinach, tomato, pumpkin, cabbage
Others: milk, bean curd

Foods To Be Avoided:

Fatty foods except butter
Stimulating foods, wine

ANEMIA

High-calorie, high-protein diet; nutritious foods with vitamins B_{12} and C, folic acid, and iron; liver and fruits to increase blood cells; restricted fat, sugar, and salt.

Allowable Foods:

Meats: liver, kidney, heart, uterus, stomach, gizzard
Vegetables: beans, spinach, cabbage, asparagus, lettuce, perilla, chrysanthemum
Fruits: peaches, apricots, raisins, grapes, apples
Others: egg yolks, oysters

Foods To Be Avoided:

Beverages: milk, coffee, tea

HEART DISEASE

Easily digested foods in small quantities, frequent meals; low-fat, low-salt diet; no spicy, stimulating foods and foods with high water content; sparse seasonings and sauces; frequent helpings of vegetables, fruits, and honey to prevent constipation.

Allowable Foods:

Meats: fish, chicken
Grains: cooked rice, bread, noodles
Vegetables: potatoes, lily root, spinach, cabbage
Fruits: grapes, peaches, loquats, bananas
Fats: butter, rape seed oil
Others: eggs, bean curd, milk, mayonnaise

Foods To Be Avoided:

Vegetables: beans, taro, arctium, turnips, napa
Aromatic and acrid foods: stimulants, aromatic foods, pepper, mustard
Beverages: carbonated drinks

GASTRIC ULCER

Nutritious, high-vitamin, low-fat diet; easily digested foods; frequent small meals; food neither very hot nor very cold, chewed carefully; no smoking.

Allowable Foods:

Meats: eggs, chicken, low-fat fish, oysters
Grains: soft cooked rice, rice gruel, noodles, bread, wheat powder
Vegetables: fully cooked, bland vegetables
Fruits
Fats: butter
Beverages: light tea, soda water, milk
Others: bean curd, milk products

Foods To Be Avoided:

Meats: conch, pork, tuna, mackerel, eel, herrings, sepia
Vegetables: arctium, bamboo, sweet potatoes, lotus root, kelp, high-fiber or hard vegetables
Stimulants: mustard, pepper, curry, cayenne pepper, coffee, wine
Others: vinegar, miso, salted foods

STOMACH DISEASE, CHRONIC GASTRITIS

Easily digested foods and fluids to prevent constipation; sufficient calories; food neither very hot nor very cold. Avoid stimulating the stomach.

Allowable Foods:

Meats: fish, shredded meat, low-fiber meat
Grains: cooked rice, rice gruel, bread
Vegetables
Dairy products: milk, cheese, butter
Bean products: beans, bean curd
Others: eggs

Foods To Be Avoided:

Vegetables: arctium, lotus root, seaweed, sweet potatoes, taro
Fats except butter, especially fried foods
Beverages: alcohol, coffee, tea, cocoa, carbonated drinks
Spices: vinegar, salt, miso
Others: pickled vegetables, salted fish, smoked fish or meat

GASTRITIS, GASTROPTOSIS

Nutritious, high-calorie diet to improve strength.

Allowable Foods:

Meats: chicken, low-fat fish
Grains: cooked rice, noodles
Dairy products: butter, milk
Others: egg yolks, cookies

Foods To Be Avoided:

Fatty foods: beef, pork, sausage, preserved meats, salted fish, vegetable oil
Low calorie foods: vegetables, fruits

DIARRHEA

Avoid easily fermented foods such as milk and honey.

Allowable Foods:

Meats: fish
Grains: rice gruel, bread
Vegetables: vegetable juice such as carrot, spinach, potato
Others: eggs, cookies, gelatinous foods

Foods To Be Avoided:

Meats: smoked or salted fish, bacon, salted meats
Grains: unpolished rice, wheat, cooked rice
Vegetables: bamboo, lotus root, seaweed, bean curd, high-fiber vegetables
Fats: all fats except butter
Others: acidic or vinegar products

CONSTIPATION

A diet to improve intestinal peristalsis.

Allowable Foods:

Meats: fish, salted or dried
Grains: unpolished rice, germinated rice, cooked wheat, buckwheat
Vegetables: spinach, turnips, potatoes, squash, pumpkin, peas, seaweed
Fruits
Fats: butter, glycerine, sesame oil, yolk oil
Spices: pepper, agar, wasabia

Foods To Be Avoided:

Meat
Eggs

GOUT

No alcohol.

Allowable Foods:

Grains
Fruits
Beverages: coffee, tea
Others: eggs, milk, cabbage

Foods To Be Avoided:

Meats: fatty meats, liver, gravy
Vegetables: spinach, beans, peas, mushrooms
Beverages: alcohol
Others: foods containing sodium, salt, soda water

ACUTE RHEUMATISM

High-protein, high-vitamin diet to improve resistance and strengthen blood vessels.

Allowable Foods:

Dairy products: cheese, butter, milk
Vegetables: cabbage, carrots, cucumbers
Fruits: oranges, apples, grapes, bananas, strawberries, tomatoes
Others: bread, eggs

Foods To Be Avoided:

Beverages: alcohol
Stimulating foods
Spices: salt

EPILEPSY

Low-protein, low-salt diet; reduced fluids; vegetarian diet to increase the body's acidity; no smoking.

Allowable Foods:

Vegetables: as many as desired
Fats: lard, sesame oil, vegetable oil, butter, fried foods
Beverages: tea, cocoa, fruit juice

Foods To Be Avoided:

Beverages: coffee, alcohol, stimulants
Spices: salt
Stimulating foods

HEMORRHOIDS

High-fat diet; foods good for constipation.

Allowable Foods:

Meats: pork
Grains: wheat
Vegetables: seaweed, beans, mushrooms, taro, high-fiber vegetables
Fruits
Dairy products: butter, cheese, milk
Beverages: beer
Others: fried foods, mayonnaise, sweets

Foods To Be Avoided:

Grains: glutinous rice cakes
Fruits: persimmons
Beverages: wine
Spices: pepper

III. DISEASES, SYMPTOMS, AND FORMULAS

ABDOMINAL PAIN

Formula of Choice:

Pinellia Combination *(Pan-hsia-hsieh-hsin-tang)* or Pinellia and Ginseng Six Combination *(Pan-hsia-liu-chun-tzu-tang)*

nausea, vomiting, resistance beneath the sternum

Alternate Formulas:

Cardamon and Fennel Formula *(An-chung-san)*

poor complexion, succussion sound beneath the sternum, persistent stomachache

Cinnamon and Peony Combination *(Kuei-chih-chia-shao-yao-tang)* or Minor Cinnamon and Peony Combination *(Hsiao-chien-chung-tang)*

gastroptosis, abdominal distention, succussion sound and gas in the abdomen, a sensation of distention in the lower abdomen, abdominal pain; for emaciated people, Minor Cinnamon and Peony Combination is advised

Peony and Licorice Combination *(Shao-yao-kan-tsao-tang)*

muscular spasms, severe abdominal pain, kidney

stones, cholelithiasis, severe intestinal colic due to dysmenorrhea

Hoelen Five Herb Formula *(Wu-ling-san)* or Ginseng and Ginger Combination *(Jen-sheng-tang)*
severe vomiting, pain in the lower abdomen

Coptis Combination *(Huang-lien-tang)*
pain between the lower sternum and umbilicus, acute gastritis

Tang-kuei and Peony Formula *(Tang-kuei-shao-yao-san)*
women with pain in the lower abdomen or abdominal pain during pregnancy

ABNORMAL URINATION

Formula of Choice:
Hoelen Five Herb Formula *(Wu-ling-san)*
rough urination due to nephritis, nephralgia, heart disease

Alternate Formulas:
Polyporus Combination *(Chu-ling-tang)*
difficult urination due to cystitis, urethritis, hematuria, painful urination

Rehmannia Eight Formula *(Pa-wei-ti-huang-wan)*
polyuria, retention of urine, incontinence due to diabetes mellitus

Capillaris Combination *(Yin-chen-hao-tang)*
thirst, oliguria, constipation, distention in the upper abdomen due to liver or biliary disease

ADENOSIS CONSTITUTION, FAULTY DEVELOPMENT IN CHILDREN

Formula of Choice:

Ginseng and Atractylodes Formula *(Sheng-ling-pai-chu-san)*

emaciation, poor complexion, anorexia, a tendency towards chronic diarrhea, chronic diarrhea, weakness during convalescence, fatigability

Alternate Formulas:

Ginseng and Astragalus Combination *(Pu-chung-i-chi-tang)*

an adenosis constitution, weakness, emaciation, a tubercular constitution

Minor Cinnamon and Peony Combination *(Hsiao-chien-chung-tang)*

weak constitution, fatigability, poor complexion, abdominal pain, palpitations, cold hands and feet, a febrile sensation, frequent urination or polyuria; also for weak children with anxiety, night crying, enuresis, chronic gastritis; a tonic

ALOPECIA AREATA

Formula of Choice:

Cinnamon and Dragon Bone Combination *(Kuei-chih-chia-lung-ku-mu-li-tang)*

hair loss, dandruff, "flushing up," fatigability

Alternate Formulas:

Major Bupleurum Combination *(Ta-chai-hu-tang)*
for people of average physical strength, fullness in the heart and constipation

Bupleurum and Peony Formula *(Chia-wei-hsiao-yao-san)*
hair loss, melasma

Bupleurum and Dragon Bone Combination *(Chai-hu-chia-lung-ku-mu-li-tang)*
anxiety, a tendency to lose hair

ANEMIA

Formula of Choice:

Ginseng and *Tang-kuei* Ten Combination *(Shih-chuan-ta-pu-tang)*
loss of strength during convalescence, pale skin, emaciation, fatigability, lassitude, anorexia, night sweats, cold hands and feet, anemia

Alternate Formulas:

Tang-kuei Four Combination *(Szu-wu-tang)*
dry skin, poor complexion, menoxenia, chills; no gastrointestinal problems; recovery after childbirth or abortion

Four Major Herb Combination *(Szu-chun-tzu-tang)* or Six Major Herb Combination *(Liu-chun-tzu-tang)*
emaciation, poor complexion, anorexia, fatigability, gastric ulcers, gastric cancer, anemia due to loss of strength

ANOREXIA

Formula of Choice:

Pinellia Combination *(Pan-hsia-hsieh-hsin-tang)* or Pinellia and Ginseng Six Combination *(Pan-hsieh-liu-chun-tzu-tang)*

distention and congestion in the stomach, anorexia, nausea, vomiting, diarrhea, soft stools or a tendency towards diarrhea

Alternate Formulas:

Six Major Herb Combination *(Liu-chun-tzu-tang)*

noticeable water stagnancy in the stomach, indigestion after meals, anorexia

Magnolia and Ginger Formula *(Ping-wei-san)*

indigestion after meals, anorexia due to a tendency towards dyspepsia

Minor Bupleurum Combination *(Hsiao-chai-hu-tang)*

the final stage of a common cold, fatigability, a bitter taste in the mouth, white tongue fur, nausea, gastritis, anorexia due to gastrointestinal weakness—especially anorexia caused by liver disorders

Astragalus and Atractylodes Combination *(Ching-su-i-chi-tang)*

sunstroke, diarrhea, general lassitude, anorexia due to the heat

Ginseng and Ginger Combination *(Jen-sheng-tang)*
weak people with anorexia; abdominal weakness, cold hands and feet, polyuria, gastrointestinal weakness, gastric weakness, diarrhea, vomiting, stomachache

Ginseng and Astragalus Combination *(Pu-chung-i-chi-tang)*
anorexia due to fatigue, lack of vitality, regression of gastrointestinal function, a weak constitution, lassitude, weakness during convalescence, night sweats

APPENDICITIS, CHRONIC

Formula of Choice:

Rhubarb and Moutan Combination *(Ta-huang-mu-tan-pi-tang)* or Cinnamon and Hoelen Formula *(Kuei-chih-fu-ling-wan)*
lower abdominal ulcers with no stimulating condition in surrounding abdominal membrane; for strong people in good health with pain in the lower abdomen, and constipation

Alternate Formula:

Bupleurum and Cinnamon Combination *(Chai-hu-kuei-chih-tang)*
first stage appendicitis, pain in the lower right abdomen

BILIARY DISEASE

Formula of Choice:

Capillaris Combination *(Yin-chen-hao-tang)*
thirst, oliguria, constipation, jaundice

BURNS

Formula of Choice:

Lithospermum Ointment *(Tzu-yun-kao)*

a topical ointment

Alternate Formulas:

Coptis and Rhubarb Combination *(San-huang-hsieh-hsin-tang)*

mild burns; mental instability, irascibility, mild fever. For long term medication, Coptis and Scute Combination *(Huang-lien-chieh-tu-tang)* is used.

Bupleurum and Dragon Bone Combination *(Chai-hu-chia lung-ku-mu-li-tang)*

palpitations, instability, excitability, thoraco-costal distress, spasms, fever

CANCER, GASTRIC

Formula of Choice:

WTTC *(Lo-shih-shu)*

a cancer therapy in Japan used in the initial stage of gastric cancer; also used to prevent relapse after surgery. Six Major Herb Combination *(Liu-chun-tzu-tang)* is given in conjunction to improve the appetite.

CATARACTS, GLAUCOMA

Formula of Choice:

Rehmannia Six Formula *(Liu-wei-ti-huang-wan)* or
Rehmannia Eight Formula *(Pa-wei-ti-huang-wan)*

geriatric cataracts, glaucoma; especially good for

weakness in the legs and feet, and pain from coldness in the loin

Alternate Formulas:

Gambir Formula *(Ko-teng-san)*

glaucoma due to hypotension; headaches

Chrysanthemum Combination *(Tzu-shen-ming-mu-tang)*

nervous exhaustion, renal weakness, weakness due to prolonged illness, weak *ch'i* and blood, aching eyes, eyestrain, fear of light

Ginseng and Ginger Combination *(Jen-sheng-tang)*

cataracts and glaucoma due to a poor gastrointestinal tract

CHEST PAIN

Formula of Choice:

Gardenia and Soja Combination *(Chih-tzu-shih-tang)* or
Coptis and Scute Combination *(Huang-lien-chieh-tu-tang)*

chest pain with thoracic distention; prevents angina pectoris

Alternate Formulas:

Minor Bupleurum Combination *(Hsiao-chai-hu-tang)* or
Bupleurum and Scute Combination *(Chai-hsien-tang)*

a sensation of pressure in the chest, chest pain while coughing

Minor Cinnamon and Peony Combination *(Hsiao-chien-chung-tang)*

chest pain due to severe pain

Tang-kuei Combination *(Tang-kuei-tang)*
cold back, gas in the upper abdomen, chest pain due to pressure in the chest

Ginseng and Ginger Combination *(Jen-sheng-tang)*
chest pain caused by digestive disorders—a stabbing pain felt from abdomen to chest

CHILDBIRTH, TONICS FOR (Before and After)

Formula of Choice:

Tang-kuei and Peony Combination *(Tang-kuei-shao-yao-san)*
a tonic for pregnant or postpartum women

Alternate Formulas:

Tang-kuei and Parsley Combination *(Pao-chan-wu-yu-fang)*
also named *Shih-san-wei* or *An-tai-yin*; vomiting of pregnancy, heavy headedness, vertigo, unstable fetal movement

Tang-kuei and Ginger Combination *(Sheng-hua-tang)*
for nutrition after childbirth; postpartum abdominal pain, abdominal pain; nourishes the blood

Dandelion Combination *(Pu-kung-ying-tang)*
insufficient milk

CHILDHOOD ASTHMA, WHOOPING COUGH

ASTHMA

Formula of Choice:

Ma-huang and Apricot Seed Combination *(Ma-hsin-kan-shih-tang)*

severe coughing, stridor, a dry throat, severe perspiration at onset; children's asthma

WHOOPING COUGH

Formula of Choice:

Minor Blue Dragon Combination *(Hsiao-ching-lung-tang)*

watery cough or cough with nasal drip; sneezing

ASTHMA AND WHOOPING COUGH

Formula of Choice:

Ophiopogon Combination *(Mai-men-tung-tang)* or

Platycodon and Fritillary Combination *(Ching-fei-tang)*

cough with ceaseless sputum, bronchitis, bronchial asthma

Alternate Formula:

Minor Bupleurum Combination with Pinellia and Magnolia Combination *(Hsiao-chai-hu-tang-chia-pan-hsia-hou-pu-tang)*

childhood anxiety, persistent cough, mental instability, anorexia, nausea

CHILLS IN WOMEN

Formula of Choice:

Tang-kuei and Peony Formula *(Tang-kuei-shao-yao-san)*
chills, anemia, fatigability

Alternate Formulas:

Cinnamon and Hoelen Formula *(Kuei-chi-fu-ling-wan)*
"flushing up," occluded blood in the lower eyelids, headaches, tinnitus, shoulder stiffness, vertigo, cardiac hyperfunction, chills, pain when pressed on the lower abdomen

Tang-kuei, Evodia, and Ginger Combination *(Tang-kuei-szu-ni-chia-wu-chu-yu-sheng-chiang-tang)*
cold hands and feet, pain in the lower limbs or abdomen when the lower limbs become cold, headaches, lower back pain, chillblains

Rehmannia Eight Formula *(Pa-wei-ti-huang-wan)*
chills in the elderly, cold hands and feet, occasional fever; polyuria, oliguria, or a sensation of residual urine

COMMON COLDS

Formula of Choice:

Pueraria Combination *(Ko-ken-tang)*
an average constitution; a common cold, headaches, fever, chills, tremors, no sweating, stiff shoulders, muscle pain, hand and shoulder pain

COUGHS

Formula of Choice:

Minor Blue Dragon Combination *(Hsiao-ching-lung-tang)*
frequent coughing, large quantities of thin sputum, bronchitis, bronchial asthma, nasal drip, rhinitis

Alternate Formulas:

***Ma-huang* and Ginkgo Combination *(Ting-chuan-tang)* or**
Apricot Seed and *Ma-huang* Combination *(Ma-hsing-kan-shih-tang)*
fever, sputum, gasping, yellowish sputum, frequent coughing, thirst, children's asthma, bronchial asthma

COMMON COLDS WITH STUFFY NOSE

Formula of Choice:

Pueraria and Magnolia Combination *(Ko-ken-tang-chia-chuan-chung-hsin-i)*
stuffy nose, nasal suppuration, chronic rhinitis

Alternate Formulas:

Bupleurum and Cinnamon Combination *(Chai-hu-kuei-chih-tang)*
prolonged, severe common cold; mild fever; fear of chills; headaches; a tendency towards vomiting

Ma-huang Combination *(Ma-huang-tang)*
strong people with fear of chills, fever, headaches, no sweating, general pain, coughing

Minor Bupleurum Combination *(Hsiao-chai-hu-tang)*
severe common cold, mild fever, chest pain, anorexia, fatigability, gastritis, gastric weakness

Pinellia and Magnolia Combination *(Pan-hsia-hou-pu-tang)*
a sensation of obstruction in the throat and esophagus, palpitations, vertigo, anxiety, mental instability, hoarseness

Ophiopogon Combination *(Mai-men-tung-tang)*
thick sputum with coughing, ceaseless sputum, dry skin, "flushing up," bronchitis, asthma

Platycodon and Fritillary Combination *(Ching-fei-tang)*
chronic coughing, frequent coughing, prolonged coughing, or coughing with copious sputum

Cinnamon Combination *(Kuei-chih-tang)*
loss of vitality with a common cold, fear of chills, fever, headaches, spontaneous sweating

Pueraria Combination with Minor Bupleurum Combination *(Ko-ken-tang-chia-hsiao-chai-hu-tang)*
headaches, nasal dryness, thirst, pain in the arms and legs, influenza, pneumonia, feverish diseases

Ma-huang and Cimicifuga Combination *(Shih-shen-tang)*
a modified formula of Pueraria Combination; fever, fear of chills, headaches, coughing, gasping, a tendency towards vomiting

Morus and Chrysanthemum Combination *(Sang-chu-yin)*
a common cold caught in subtropical zones and tropical zones with warm winds

Ma-huang, Aconite, and Asarum Combination *(Ma-huang-hsi-hsin-fu-tzu-tang)*
weak and elderly people with chills

Hoelen and Schizandra Combination *(Ling-kan-chiang-wei-hsin-hsia-jen-tang)*
chronic symptoms, geriatric weakness, frequent urination, chills, edema, anemia

Bupleurum and Pueraria Combination *(Chai-ko-chieh-chi-tang)*
severe common cold, headaches, nasal dryness, thirst, annoying pain in the arms and legs, a quick pulse

Cyperus and Perilla Formula *(Hsiang-su-san)*
for people with a poor gastrointestinal tract with a common cold; neurosis

Ma-huang and Morus Formula *(Hua-kai-san)*
gasping, coughing, "flushing up," annoyance in the chest, convulsions in the neck and back, nasal obstruction

Ma-huang and Magnolia Combination *(Shen-mi-tang)*
asthma, a severe cough, dyspnea, children's asthma, bronchial asthma, bronchitis; suitable for long term use

CONJUNCTIVAL CONGESTION AND HEMORRHAGE

Formula of Choice:

Coptis and Rhubarb Combination *(San-huang-hsieh-hsin-*

tang) or Coptis and Scute Combination *(Huang-lien-chieh-tu-tang)*

eye congestion or hemorrhage due to "flushing up," excitability, instability, insomnia. Coptis and Scute Combination is used if no constipation occurs.

Alternate Formula:

Tang-kuei and Gardenia Combination *(Wen-ching-yin)*

poor complexion, "flushing up," persistent congestion, conjunctival hemorrhage

CONSTIPATION, HABITUAL

Formula of Choice:

Coptis and Rhubarb Combination *(San-huang-hsieh-hsin-tang)*

for vigorous people with a tendency to "flush up," "liver fire," mental instability, anxiety, constipation

Alternate Formulas:

Apricot Seed and Linum Formula *(Ma-tzu-jen-wan)*

for elderly and weak people with dry skin and habitual constipation

Major Bupleurum Combination *(Ta-chai-hu-tang)*

for people of sturdy build and good appetite with frequent constipation, thoraco-costal distress, and abdominal distention; also for gastritis, headaches due to hypertension, shoulder stiffness

Siler and Platycodon Formula *(Fang-feng-tung-sheng-san)*
for people of obese constitution with habitual constipation but without thoraco-costal distress

Minor Rhubarb Combination *(Hsiao-cheng-chi-tang)* or Major Rhubarb Combination *(Ta-cheng-chi-tang)*
constipation with abdominal distention around the umbilicus

Minor Cinnamon and Peony Combination *(Hsiao-chien-chung-tang)*
constipation in children

Tang-kuei and Peony Combination *(Tang-kuei-shao-yao-san)*
constipation during pregnancy which usually causes difficult delivery

Bupleurum and Peony Formula *(Chia-wei-hsiao-yao-san)*
for women with constipation caused by climacteric and autonomic nerve disorders

CONTUSIONS (Bruises)

Formula of Choice:

Cinnamon and Hoelen Formula *(Kuei-chih-fu-ling-wan)*
poor blood circulation, interior hemorrhaging, or bleeding due to fluxion of the wound

Alternate Formulas:

Persica and Rhubarb Combination *(Tao-ho-cheng-chi-tang)*

subepidermal hemorrhage due to swelling after bruising, severe pain, constipation, excitability

Coptis and Rhubarb Combination *(San-huang-hsieh-hsin-tang)*

excitability, facial "flushing up," hemorrhage due to an accident

Musk and Catechu Formula *(Chi-li-san)*

a traditional formula in China for contusions, occluded blood, stagnancy, and general pain

COSMETICS -- FOR ACNE, FRECKLES, MELASMA (Chloasma), WARTS

Formula of Choice:

Siler Combination *(Ching-shang-fang-feng-tang)*

acne due to stagnant fever in the face and neck; facial redness, eye congestion, facial tinea alba. To improve skin, 1g of coix is added. If constipation occurs, 0.5-1.0g of rhubarb is added.

Alternate Formulas:

Tang-kuei and Peony Formula *(Tang-kuei-shao-yao-san)*

chills, a weak constitution, pale complexion, fatigability, pigmentation around the eyes and nose such as freckles and melasma. More efficacious when associated with coix.

Cinnamon and Hoelen Formula *(Kuei-chih-fu-ling-wan)*

for people with strength who sometimes have lower abdominal pain, stiff shoulders, vertigo, heavy headedness, "flushing up," climacteric disorders, menstrual irregularities, freckles, melasma

Bupleurum and Peony Formula *(Chia-wei-hsiao-yao-san)*

for women past middle age with a weak constitution, anxiety, mental instability, easily fatigued arms and legs, and a tendency towards constipation; also menstrual irregularities, dysmenorrhea, climacteric disorders, chills

Coix Decoction *(I-yi-jen-chien)*

warts; decoct 30.0g of coix with 1.0-5.0g of licorice

CYSTITIS, URETHRITIS, PROSTATOMEGALY

Formula of Choice:

Lotus Seed Combination *(Ching-hsin-lien-tzu-yin)*

general lassitude, a weak gastrointestinal tract, a dry mouth, difficult urination, turbid urine, a sensation of residual urine, frequent urination, painful urination, chronic gonorrhea, pyelitis, renal tuberculosis, leukorrhea, involuntary emissions, sexual fears, prostatomegaly, cystitis, urethritis

Alternate Formulas:

Rehmannia Eight Formula *(Pa-wei-ti-huang-wan)* or
Rehmannia Six Formula *(Liu-wei-ti-huang-wan)*

a Lotus Seed Combination conformation—lower back pain, eye fatigability, reduction of eyesight, impotence, chronic nephritis, renal atrophy, bedwetting. Rehmannia Six Formula is used for children and people of average constitution.

Polyporus Combination *(Chu-ling-tang)*
thirst, oliguria, difficult urination, painful urination, a sensation of residual urine, urethral calculi, vesical calculi, gonorrhea

Tang-kuei and Peony Formula *(Tang-kuei-shao-yao-san)*
for women of poor physical strength with frequent urination and chills, and pain in the lower abdomen

Gentiana Combination *(Lung-tan-hsieh-kan-tang)*
for people of average physical strength with painful urination due to tense lower abdominal muscles, a sensation of residual urine, turbid urine and stuttering urination, and leukorrhea

DIABETES MELLITUS

Formula of Choice:

Rehmannia Six Formula *(Liu-wei-ti-huang-wan)*
fatigability, oliguria or polyuria, thirst, vertigo, tinnitus, involuntary emissions, weakness and atrophy of the lumbus and knee, edema, itching

Alternate Formulas:

Rehmannia Eight Formula *(Pa-wei-ti-huang-wan)*
for people weaker than the Rehmannia Six *(Liu-wei-ti-huang-wan)* conformation with cold arms and legs, lower back pain, pain in the legs and feet, presbyopia, itching, difficult urination, frequent urination, edema

Ginseng and Gypsum Combination *(Pai-hu-chia-jen-sheng-tang)*
a dry mouth, severe thirst, the initial stage of diabetes mellitus, frequent urination, fatigability

Four Major Herb Combination *(Szu-chun-tzu-tang)*
emaciation, a poor complexion, anorexia, fatigability, a weak gastrointestinal tract

Siler and Platycodon Formula *(Fang-feng-tung-sheng-san)*
for strong people; prevents diabetes mellitus

Major Bupleurum Combination with dried rehmannia *(Ta-chai-hu-tang-chia-kan-ti-huang)*
for people of average physical strength with thoraco-costal distress, constipation, and shoulder stiffness

Minor Bupleurum Combination with dried rehmannia *(Hsiao-chai-hu-tang-chia-kan-ti-huang)*
weak conformation, thirst, fatigability, anorexia, thoraco-costal distress

DIARRHEA

Formula of Choice:

Pinellia Combination *(Pan-hsia-hsieh-hsin-tang)* or Pinellia and Ginseng Six Combination *(Pan-hsieh-liu-chun-tzu-tang)*
nausea, vomiting, anorexia, gas, soft stools, a tendency towards diarrhea, fermentative diarrhea, dyspepsia, nervous gastritis, gastric weakness

Alternate Formulas:

Six Major Herb Combination *(Liu-chun-tzu-tang)*
diarrhea, gastric weakness, anorexia, a feeling of distention and stagnation in the stomach, dyspepsia,

fatigability, gastritis, gastroptosis, stomachache, vomiting

Hoelen Five Herb Formula *(Wu-ling-san)*
children's watery diarrhea, thirst with abdominal pain, vomiting, nausea, headaches, edema, sunstroke, tenesmus

Cinnamon and Peony Combination *(Kuei-chih-chia-shao-yao-tang)*
diarrhea with abdominal pain, abdominal distention, abdominal pain due to tenesmus

Pueraria, Coptis, and Scute Combination ***(Ko-ken-huang-lien-huang-chin-tang)***
bacterial diarrhea, diarrhea due to fever, distention below the sternum, stiff shoulders, acute gastritis, stomatitis, inflammation of the tongue, insomnia

Bupleurum and Cinnamon Combination ***(Chai-hu-kuei-chih-tang)***
diarrhea caused by tension, usually with abdominal pain

Vitality Combination *(Chen-wu-tang)*
geriatric and weak people with chronic diarrhea and abdominal pain

Pinellia and Ginger Combination *(Sheng-chiang-hsieh-hsin-tang)* or Pinellia Combination *(Pan-hsia-hsieh-hsin-tang)*
distention and hardening beneath the heart,

anorexia, gas, diarrhea, nausea, vomiting, occasional abdominal pain

DRY MOUTH AND THIRST

Formula of Choice:

Hoelen Five Herb Formula *(Wu-ling-san)*

thirst, oliguria; thirst due to stomach, intestinal, liver, and kidney disorders

Alternate Formulas:

Rehmannia Six Formula *(Liu-wei-ti-huang-wan)* or
Rehmannia Eight Formula *(Pa-wei-ti-huang-wan)*

thirst and polyuria due to diabetes mellitus

Ginseng and Gypsum Combination *(Pai-hu-chia-jen-sheng-tang)*

the initial stage of diabetes mellitus; thirst due to high fever or fever of unknown cause

Minor Bupleurum Combination *(Hsiao-chai-hu-tang)*

thirst due to pyelitis; pleuritis, pulmonary tuberculosis; mild fever, dry mouth and tongue, annoying fever in the hands and feet. More effective if rehmannia is added.

EDEMA

Formula of Choice:

Hoelen Five Herb Formula *(Wu-ling-san)*

edema with thirst and oliguria

Alternate Formulas:

Stephania and Ginseng Combination *(Mu-fang-chi-tang)*
edema due to heart disease; edema with oliguria, stridor, dry mouth, split tongue

Rehmannia Eight Formula *(Pa-wei-ti-huang-wan)*
edema due to nephritis, kidney disease and chronic disease; especially edema in the lower body

Tang-kuei and Peony Formula *(Tang-kuei-shao-yao-san)* or Cinnamon and Hoelen Formula
edema during pregnancy or after childbirth. For occluded blood, Cinnamon and Hoelen Formula is advised.

Capillaris Combination *(Yin-chen-hao-tang)*
usually given with Minor Bupleurum Combination *(Hsiao-chai-hu-tang)* for edema due to liver disorders

Stephania and Astragalus Combination *(Fang-chi-huang-chi-tang)*
edema in the lower body

Ginseng and Akebia Combination *(Pu-chung-chi-shih-tang)*
edema and general weakness

Hoelen and Alisma Combination *(Feng-hsiao-tang)*
edema due to ascites

ESOPHAGOSTENOSIS, NERVOUS

Formula of Choice:

Pinellia and Magnolia Combination *(Pan-hsia-hou-pu-tang)*

sensation of obstruction in the throat, palpitations, vertigo, belching, mental instability, vomiting of pregnancy, hoarseness

Alternate Formulas:

Evodia Combination *(Wu-chu-yu-tang)*

headaches, chills, severe nausea, vomiting, hiccoughs

Pinellia and Gardenia Combination *(Li-ke-tang)*

esophagostenosis, dysphagia

EYE FATIGUE

Formula of Choice:

Atractylodes and Hoelen Combination *(Ling-kuei-chu-kan-tang)*

vertigo, dizziness upon standing, palpitations, oliguria, heavy headedness, "flushing up," gasping, anxiety, neurosis

Alternate Formulas:

Bupleurum and Dragon Bone Combination *(Chai-hu-chia-lung-ku-mu-li-tang)*

eye ache, loss of eyesight due to neural fatigue

Bupleurum and Peony Formula *(Chia-wei-hsiao-yao-san)*

eye fatigue due to female problems

Minor Bupleurum Combination and Hoelen and Atractylodes Combination *(Hsiao-chai-hu-tang-ho-ling-kuei-chu-kan-tang)*

eye fatigue due to general fatigue

FEVER AND FEAR OF CHILLS

Formula of Choice:

Pueraria Combination *(Ko-ken-tang)*

fear of chills, fever, shoulder stiffness, absence of sweating

Alternate Formulas:

Bupleurum and Cinnamon Combination *(Chai-hu-kuei-chih-tang)*

fever, a weak pulse, night sweats; especially for a severe common cold

Minor Bupleurum Combination *(Hsiao-chai-hu-tang)*

anorexia, fatigability, bitter taste in the mouth, a sticky mouth, white tongue fur

Major Bupleurum Combination *(Ta-chai-hu-tang)*

for strong people with thoraco-costal distress, swelling and full abdominal force, and constipation; especially for fevers due to cholecystitis and hepatitis

Bupleurum Formula *(I-kan-san)*

fever of unknown cause, anxiety, fever in debilitated children

FRIGIDITY

Formula of Choice:

Cinnamon and Dragon Bone Combination *(Kuei-chih-chia-lung-ku-mu-li-tang)*

weak constitution, fatigability, excitability, palpitations and hyperfunction around the umbilicus, neurosis, insomnia, "flushing up," vertigo, loss of hair, headaches, tinnitus, night sweats

Alternate Formulas:

Bupleurum and Peony Formula *(Chia-wei-hsiao-yao-san)*
weakness of the hands and feet, fatigability, headaches, vertigo, insomnia, irritability

***Tang-kuei,* Evodia, and Ginger Combination** *(Tang-kuei-szu-ni-chia-wu-chu-yu-sheng-chiang-tang)*
cold hands and feet, distention and fullness in the chest, nausea, lower back pain, abdominal pain

Rehmannia Eight Formula *(Pa-wei-ti-huang-wan)*
weakness, fatigability, polyuria, oliguria, a dry mouth, insomnia, gasping, cold hands and feet, tinnitus

FRIGORISM (Effects of prolonged exposure to cold)

Formula of Choice:

Tang-kuei and Peony Formula *(Tang-kuei-shao-yao-san)*
anemia, chills, fatigability

Alternate Formula:

Tang-kuei, Evodia, and Ginger Combination *(Tang-kuei-szu-ni-chia-wu-chu-yu-sheng-chiang-tang)*
cold hands and feet, cold legs, pain in the legs or lower abdomen with headaches, pain in the lower abdomen, lower back pain

GASTRICISM, DUODENAL ULCERS, STOMACHACHES, GASTRIC SPASMS

Formula of Choice:

Pinellia Combination *(Pan-hsia-hsieh-hsin-tang)* or Pinellia and Ginseng Six Combination *(Pan-hsieh-liu-chun-tzu-tang)*

nausea, vomiting, anorexia, gas, dyspepsia, gastritis

Alternate Formulas:

Cardamon and Fennel Formula *(An-chung-san)*

emaciation with a tendency toward flaccid abdominal muscles, stomachache, abdominal pain, vomiting gastric acid, belching, anorexia

Six Major Herb Combination *(Liu-chun-tzu-tang)*

maintains health; a feeling of distention and pressure in the stomach, weak gastrointestinal tract, stomachache due to fatigue

Bupleurum and Cinnamon Combination *(Chai-hu-kuei-chih-tang)*

a weak constitution, anorexia, anxiety, **appendicitis** with abdominal pain, gastric ulcers, gastric spasms

GASTRICISM, GENERAL

Formula of Choice:

Pinellia Combination *(Pan-hsia-hsieh-hsin-tang)*or Pinellia and Ginseng Six Combination *(Pan-hsia-liu-chun-tzu-tang)*

stagnancy beneath the sternum, occasional nausea, vomiting, anorexia, gas, soft stools or a tendency toward diarrhea; also good for acute and chronic gastroenteritis, fermentative diarrhea, dyspepsia, gastroptosis, nervous gastritis, a weak stomach, drunkenness, belching, vomiting of bile, stomatitis, neurosis

Alternate Formulas:

Magnolia and Ginger Formula ***(Ping-wei-san)***
for a somewhat firm conformation with stomach stagnancy, dyspepsia, anorexia, abdominal distention, stagnancy beneath the heart, gas following meals, diarrhea, acute and chronic gastritis, and a weak stomach

Cardamon and Fennel Formula ***(An-chung-san)***
weakness, emaciation with a tendency toward abdominal flaccidity; also for stomachaches, abdominal pain, vomiting gastric acid, belching, anorexia, nausea, nervous gastritis, gastric weakness, pain from gastric spasms

Hoelen Five Herb Formula *(Wu-ling-san)*
acute gastroenteritis, thirst, vomiting of gastric acid, oliguria, watery diarrhea, hangover, nausea, vomiting, abdominal pain, headache, edema, sunstroke

Six Major Herb Combination *(Liu-chun-tzu-tang)*
a weak gastrointestinal tract, anorexia, fatigue, gastric stagnancy, cold hands and feet due to anemia, gastritis, gastric weakness, gastroptosis, dyspepsia, stomachache, vomiting

Ginseng and Ginger Combination *(Li-chung-tang)* or *(Jen-sheng-tang)*

cold hands and feet, poor complexion, polyuria, gastric weakness, diarrhea, vomiting, stomachache

Evodia Combination *(Wu-chu-yu-tang)*

distention below the sternum, cold hands and feet, retching with a headache, hiccoughs, gastrosia

Coptis Combination *(Huang-lien-tang)*

a feeling of pressure or stagnancy in the stomach; anorexia; acute gastritis; hangover; stomatitis; vomiting of gastric acid; nausea; thick, white fur on the tongue

GASTROPTOSIS

Formula of Choice:

Pinellia Combination *(Pan-hsia-hsieh-hsin-tang)* or Pinellia and Ginseng Six Combination *(Pan-hsieh-liu-chun-tzu-tang)*

a weak constitution; distention below the sternum, nausea, vomiting, anorexia, gas, soft stools or a tendency towards diarrhea; also acute and chronic gastroenteritis, fermentative diarrhea, dyspepsia, nervous gastritis, gastric weakness, hangover, belching, stomatitis, neurosis

Alternate Formulas:

Pinellia and Magnolia Combination *(Pan-hsia-hou-pu-tang)*

for multiparous women with a flaccid abdomen, a feeling of pressure and distention in the stomach, abdominal pain with heavy headedness and insomnia, mental instability, blocked *ch'i*, palpitations, vertigo, and nervous gastritis with belching

Ginseng and Astragalus Combination *(Pu-chung-i-chi-tang)*
lack of vitality, a weak gastrointestinal tract, fatigability; improves weakness and prolapse of the stomach and intestines

Six Major Herb Combination *(Liu-chun-tzu-tang)*
a weak constitution, anorexia; maintains health

HEADACHE

Formula of Choice:

Cnidium and Tea Formula *(Chuan-chiung-cha-tiao-san)*
common cold, headache, women's habitual headache caused by occluded blood

Alternate Formulas:

Pueraria Combination *(Ko-ken-tang)*
headache with shoulder stiffness from front to back

Bupleurum and Peony Formula *(Chia-wei-hsiao-yao-san)*
headache in women due to occluded blood; "flushing up," vertigo, shoulder stiffness, heavy headedness, menoxenia

Gambir Formula *(Kou-teng-san)*
headache due to hypertension

Pinellia and Atractylodes Combination *(Pan-hsia-pai-chu-tang)*

fatigability, headache with vertigo

Cinnamon and Ginseng Combination *(Kuei-chih-jen-sheng-tang)*

headache due to gastrointestinal weakness, gastroptosis, gastric weakness

Evodia Combination *(Wu-chu-yu-tang)*

severe paroxysmal headache with vomiting

Ma-huang*, Asarum, and Aconite Combination *(Ma-huang-hsi-hsin-fu-tzu-tang)

headache with chills in elderly and emaciated people

Hoelen Five Herb Formula *(Wu-ling-san)*

headache with thirst and oliguria

HEART DISEASE

Formula of Choice:

Bupleurum and Dragon Bone Combination *(Chai-hu-chia-lung-ku-mu-li-tang)*

cardiac hyperfunction, gasping, thoraco-costal distress, mental instability, anxiety, insomnia, paroxysmal cardiac hyperfunction, valvular disease, heart failure, angina pectoris, myocardial infarction

Alternate Formulas:

Atractylodes and Hoelen Combination *(Ling-kuei-chu-kan-tang)*

vertigo upon standing, palpitations, gasping, heavy headedness, headaches, dizziness, anxiety, neurosis, nervous cardiac hyperfunction, a weak heart, tinnitus, insomnia

Baked Licorice Combination *(Chih-kan-tsao-tang)*
palpitations, gasping, loss of body strength, fatigability, dry skin, thirst, annoying fever in the hands and feet, cardiac hyperfunction, a knotty or irregular pulse

Stephania and Ginseng Combination *(Mu-fang-chi-tang)*
gasping, stridor, oliguria, edema, distention and hardening beneath the heart, dry mouth; also endocarditis and valvular disease

Areca and Evodia Combination *(Pien-chih-hsin-chi-yin)*
oliguria, edema, palpitations, gasping, heavy headedness, blocked *ch'i*. Used when Stephania and Ginseng Combination fails.

Siler and Platycodon Formula *(Fang-feng-tung-sheng-san)*
for people of obese build with heart disease who gasp badly after slight exertion

Tang-kuei and Peony Formula *(Tang-kuei-shao-yao-san)*
for people of poor physical strength; anemia, chills, fatigability with heavy headedness, tinnitus, palpitations, vertigo, edema, cardiac weakness with shoulder stiffness

HEMORRHAGE OF GASTROINTESTINAL SYSTEM

Formula of Choice:

Coptis and Scute Combination *(Huang-lien-chieh-tu-tang)* or Coptis and Rhubarb Combination *(San-huang-hsieh-hsin-tang)*

hemoptysis due to a gastric ulcer, duodenal ulcers. For constipation, the latter formula is recommended.

Alternate Formulas:

Tang-kuei and Evodia Combination *(Wen-ching-tang)*

metrorrhagia during menopause, fever in the hands and feet, annoying fever, dry mouth and lips, coldness in the loins, abdominal pain

Ginseng and Longan Combination *(Kuei-pi-tang)*

weak constitution; poor complexion with anemia; insomnia, amnesia, cardiac hyperfunction, mental instability, neurosis

Cinnamon and Hoelen Formula *(Kuei-chih-fu-ling-wan)* or Persica and Rhubarb Combination *(Tao-ho-cheng-chi-tang)*

habitual spontaneous abortions, persistent hemorrhaging due to uterine myomatosis

Polyporus Combination *(Chu-ling-tang)*

hemorrhaging of the bladder or urethra with painful urination, frequent urination, oliguria, and a sensation of residual urine

Ginseng Combination *(Tu-sheng-tang)*

sudden severe hemorrhage

HEMORRHAGE OF RESPIRATORY SYSTEM

Formula of Choice:

Ophiopogon Combination *(Mai-men-tung-tang)* or
Platycodon and Fritillary Combination *(Ching-fei-tang)*

bloody sputum, coughing with ceaseless sputum

HEMORRHAGE FROM WOMEN'S DISEASES

Formula of Choice:

Gelatin and *Tang-kuei* Combination *(Chung-kuei-chiao-ai-tang)*

postpartum hemorrhage, hemorrhoidal bleeding, anemia, hemorrhage in the lower abdomen, uterine bleeding during pregnancy, metrorrhagia, renal hemorrhage of unknown cause, hematuria

HEMORRHOIDS

Formula of Choice:

Cimicifuga Combination *(I-tzu-tang)*

hard stools, constipation, hemorrhoidal bleeding, pain, anal fissures, the initial stage of a hernia. For severe pain, licorice is added; Lithospermum Ointment *(Tzu-yun-kao)* is used as a topical ointment.

Alternate Formulas:

Cimicifuga Combination and *Tang-kuei* Four Combination *(I-tzu-tang-ho-szu-wu-tang)*

general weakness due to hemorrhoidal hemorrhage

Cimicifuga Combination with Gelatin and *Tang-kuei* Combination *(I-tzu-tang-ho-chung-kuei-chiao-ai-tang)* persistent hemorrhoidal hemorrhaging, a tendency towards anemia

Ginseng and Astragalus Combination *(Pu-chung-i-chi-tang)*

general weakness, fear of chills, poor complexion

HERNIA

Formula of Choice:

Cinnamon and Peony Combination *(Kuei-chih-chia-shao-yao-tang)*

abdominal distention, abdominal pain from a hernia

Alternate Formula:

Major Zanthoxylum Combination *(Ta-chien-chung-tang)*

gastric weakness, vomiting, anorexia, a cold abdomen, abdominal distention, abdominal pain

HEPATOPATHY

Formula of Choice:

Minor Bupleurum Combination *(Hsiao-chai-hu-tang)*

a bitter taste in the mouth, white tongue fur, a dry throat, fatigability, anorexia, a feeling of pressure in the chest, mild fever

HEPATOPATHY, JAUNDICE, OR CHOLELITHIASIS

Formula of Choice:

Major Bupleurum Combination *(Ta-chai-hu-tang)*

for muscular people of average physical strength with

a tendency towards constipation, pain in the liver when pressed, constipation, thoraco-costal distress, fatigability, gastritis, hypertension with complications of shoulder stiffness and headache, obesity

Alternate Formulas:

Bupleurum and Cinnamon Combination *(Chai-hu-kuei-chih-tang)*

severe pain due to cholelithiasis and cholecystitis, pancreatitis; may be taken continuously after the disappearance of pain

Bupleurum, Cinnamon, and Ginger Combination ***(Chai-hu-kuei-chih-kan-chiang-tang)***

for people of little physical strength with chills, anemia, palpitations, gasping, somnolence, hepatitis, cholecystitis, acute nephritis, nephropathy, severe fatigability

Bupleurum and Peony Formula *(Chia-wei-hsiao-yao-san)*

for women with weak constitutions, fatigability, mental instability, insomnia, the initial stage of cirrhosis without jaundice, and ascites

Peony and Licorice Combination *(Shao-yao-kan-tsao-tang)*

for the onset of cholelithiasis; also for pain such as in the arms and legs, spasms, gastric spasms, abdominal pain, colic due to a kidney stone, cystalgia due to muscular spasms

HICCOUGHS

Formula of Choice:

Evodia Combination *(Wu-chu-yu-tang)*

a submerged pulse, distention below the sternum, cold hands and feet

Alternate Formula:

Kaki Combination *(Shih-ti-tang)*

hiccoughs caused by chilling of the stomach

HOARSENESS

Formula of Choice:

Ophiopogon Combination ***(Mai-men-tung-tang)***

severe cough, a dry or burning sensation in the throat

Alternate Formula:

Gasping Formula ***(Hsiang-sheng-po-ti-wan)***

hoarseness due to excessive singing and talking

HORDEOLUM, KERATITIS

Formula of Choice:

Pueraria Combination *(Ko-ken-tang)*

the initial stage—reddening, swelling, pain, headache, fear of chills, fever. For constipation, rhubarb is added or Cnidium and Rhubarb Formula *(Chiang-huang-san)* is used.

Alternate Formulas:

Atractylodes Combination *(Yueh-pi-chia-chu-tang)*
for the initial stage of keratitis in people of normal physical strength with congestion, reddening, swelling, erosion of the blephara, pain, suppuration, tearing

Bupleurum and Schizonepeta Combination *(Shih-wei-pai-tu-tang)* **or Platycodon and** *Chih-shih* **Formula** *(Pai-nung-san)*
more effective if platycodon is present; for hordeolum with a tendency towards suppuration

Minor Blue Dragon Combination *(Hsiao-ching-lung-tang)*
severe tearing due to conjunctival inflammation and congestion

Gardenia and Vitex Combination *(Hsi-kan-ming-mu-tang)*
for people of normal physical strength with ulcers in the keratoderma, fear of light, and aching eyes; keratitis. Used after acute inflammation has been alleviated.

HYPERHIDROSIS, NIGHT SWEATS

Formula of Choice:

Ginseng and Astragalus Combination *(Pu-chung-i-chi-tang)* or Astragalus Combination *(Huang-chi-chien-chung-tang)*
for people lacking vitality and of weak constitution with fatigability, anorexia, and night sweats due to weakness during convalescence

Alternate Formulas:

Stephania and Astragalus Combination *(Fang-chi-huang-chi-tang)*
hyperhidrosis during the summer in people with soft muscles, white skin, and obese constitutions

Hoelen Five Herb Formula *(Wu-ling-san)*
severe thirst, oliguria

Bupleurum and Dragon Bone Combination *(Chai-hu-chia-lung-ku-mu-li-tang)*
nervousness, perspiration

Bupleurum and Peony Formula *(Chia-wei-hsiao-yao-san)*
for women of weak constitution with anxiety, fatigability, and perspiration

Aconite and G.L. Combination *(Szu-ni-tang)*
fatigability, a sensation of hard pressure in the chest and abdomen, perspiration, cold sweat, collapse

Cinnamon and Astragalus Combination *(Kuei-chih-chia-huang-chi-tang)*
for people of weak constitution who catch colds with hyperhidrosis easily

HYPERTENSION AND ARTERIOSCLEROSIS

Formula of Choice:

Coptis and Rhubarb Combination *(San-huang-hsieh-hsin-tang)*
for people of average physical strength; red complexion, constitution prone to apoplexy, anxiety,

"flushing up," shoulder stiffness, tinnitus, heavy headedness, a tendency towards constipation. If there is no proneness for constipation, Coptis and Scute Combination is used *(Huang-lien-chieh-tu-tang)*.

Alternate Formulas:

Major Bupleurum Combination *(Ta-chai-hu-tang)*

for strong people of muscular build with a sensation of pressure in the chest, shoulder stiffness, and constipation

Bupleurum and Dragon Bone Combination *(Chai-hu-chia-lung-ku-mu-li-tang)*

for people who appear healthy, like the Major Bupleurum *(Ta-chai-hu-tang)* conformation, but have palpitations, vertigo, insomnia, neurosis exhibiting mental instability and terror, and gasping

Siler and Platycodon Formula *(Fang-feng-tung-sheng-san)*

for obese people of average physical strength with a short neck and big, swollen abdomen with palpitations, shoulder stiffness, headaches, and a tendency towards constipation; also prevents hypertension

Gambir Formula *(Kou-teng-san)*

morning headaches, migraines, tinnitus, vertigo, blocked *ch'i*, shoulder stiffness, shoulder and back spasms, loss of memory; mostly for people with hypertension due to cerebroarteriosclerosis, hypertension after middle age, or persistent headaches

Tang-kuei and Gambir Combination *(Chi-wu-chiang-hsia-tang)*
prolonged illness, loss of physical strength, a tendency towards nephrosclerosis; proteinuria, heavy headedness, shoulder stiffness, tinnitus

Rehmannia Eight Formula *(Pa-wei-ti-huang-wan)*
a dry mouth, fatigability, lower back pain, hypertension in the elderly with frequent urination

Ma-huang and Ginseng Combination *(Hsu-ming-tang)*
dyskinesia, dysphonia due to apoplexy; neuroparalysis, monoplegia

Atractylodes and Hoelen Combination *(Ling-kuei-chu-kan-tang)*
vertigo, dizziness, palpitations, headaches, gasping

HYPERTHYROIDISM

Formula of Choice:

Baked Licorice Combination *(Chih-kan-tsao-tang)*
loss of vitality, fatigability, palpitations, gasping, irregular pulse

Alternate Formulas:

Bupleurum and Dragon Bone Combination *(Chai-hu-chia-lung-ku-mu-li-tang)*
mental instability, palpitations, insomnia

Bupleurum and Peony Formula *(Chia-wei-hsiao-yao-san)*
mental instability, menoxenia, heavy headedness, shoulder stiffness, "flushing up," insomnia, vertigo, palpitations, tinnitus, cold feet

Pinellia and Magnolia Combination *(Pan-hsia-hou-pu-tang)*

mental instability, palpitations, insomnia; gastrointestinal problems occurring after using Baked Licorice Combination *(Chih-kan-tsao-tang)*

HYPOTENSION

Formula of Choice:

Ginseng and Astragalus Combination *(Pu-chung-i-chi-tang)*

poor gastrointestinal tract, a tendency toward anemia, fatigability, anorexia; strengthens the body and nourishes the blood

Alternate Formulas:

Tang-kuei and Peony Formula *(Tang-kuei-shao-yao-san)*

for people of a chillphobic constitution with anemia, fatigability, and a pale and blue complexion; nourishes the blood, warms the body, raises blood pressure

Atractylodes and Hoelen Combination *(Ling-kuei-chu-kan-tang)*

vertigo, dizziness, palpitations, gasping. *Tang-kuei* and Peony Formula *(Tang-kuei-shao-yao-san)* may be used in conjunction with this formula for anemic people of a chillphobic constitution.

Vitality Combination *(Chen-wu-tang)*
fatigability, diarrhea, cold hands and feet, vertigo, weakness

Pinellia and Gastrodia Combination *(Pan-hsia-pai-chu-tien-ma-tang)*
gastroptosis, gastric weakness, fatigability, cold hands and feet, vertigo, headaches, nausea, somnolence after meals

IMPROVING AND ENHANCING BODY STRENGTH

Formula of Choice:

Ginseng Nutritive Combination *(Jen-sheng-yang-yung-tang)*
lassitude, anorexia, night sweats, cold hands and feet, weakness during convalescence, anemia

Alternate Formulas:

Ginseng and *Tang-kuei* Ten Combination *(Shih-chuan-ta-pu-tang)*
a weak conformation, severe anemia, anorexia, cold hands and feet, night sweats, weakness during convalescence, lassitude

Ginseng and Astragalus Combination *(Pu-chung-i-chi-tang)*
a weak constitution with weakness, a poor gastrointestinal tract, fatigability, weakness during convalescence, anorexia, night sweats

Rehmannia Six Formula *(Liu-wei-ti-huang-wan)*
fatigue, oliguria or polyuria, occasional extreme thirst, weakness in the loins and knees, difficult urination, frequent urination, edema, itching

Rehmannia Eight Formula *(Pa-wei-ti-huang-wan)*
Rehmannia Six Formula symptoms plus cold arms and legs, pain in the legs and feet, lower back pain, numb hands and feet, presbyopia, itching

Minor Cinnamon and Peony Combination *(Hsiao-chien-chung-tang)*
a weak constitution (child or adult), fatigability, poor complexion, cold hands and feet, frequent or copious urination, bedwetting, anxiety, chronic gastroenteritis

Ginseng and Atractylodes Formula *(Sheng-ling-pai-chu-san)*
emaciation, poor complexion, anorexia, chronic diarrhea, weakness during convalescence, lassitude

INFERTILITY, HABITUAL ABORTION

Formula of Choice:

Tang-kuei and Peony Formula *(Tang-kuei-shao-yao-san)*
chills, a tendency toward anemia

Alternate Formulas:

Bupleurum and Peony Formula *(Chia-wei-hsiao-yao-san)*
menoxenia, "flushing up," headaches, vertigo, palpitations, anxiety, inability to conceive

Tang-kuei and Evodia Combination *(Wen-ching-tang)*
chills, menoxenia, dry mouth and lips, inability to conceive, annoying fever in the hands

Cinnamon and Hoelen Formula *(Kuei-chih-fu-ling-wan)*
for women who are not pregnant and have scanty and delayed menstruation or dysmenorrhea

Ginseng and *Tang-kuei* Ten Combination *(Shih-chuan-ta-pu-tang)*
for women of weak constitution with severe anemia, emaciation, anorexia, and fatigability

IRITIS

Formula of Choice:

Pueraria Combination *(Ko-ken-tang)*
the initial stage of any eye disease

Alternate Formulas:

Cinnamon and Hoelen Formula *(Kuei-chih-fu-ling-wan)* or Persica and Rhubarb Combination *(Tao-ho-cheng-chi-tang)*
for women of normal physical strength with "flushing up," cold feet, and gynecological diseases

Tang-kuei and Peony Formula *(Tang-kuei-shao-yao-san)*
for people of relatively poor physical strength with persistent eye disease but no serious congestion

JAUNDICE

Formula of Choice:

Capillaris Combination *(Yin-chen-hao-tang)*
the initial stage of acute hepatitis with anorexia, constipation, oliguria, fever

Alternate Formulas:

Capillaris and Hoelen Formula *(Yin-chen-wu-ling-san)*
thirst, oliguria, jaundice

Major Bupleurum Combination *(Ta-chai-hu-tang)*
thirst, dysuria, thoraco-costal distress

Ginseng and Ginger Combination *(Jen-sheng-tang)*
weak constitution, jaundice, abdominal flaccidity, anorexia, diarrhea, vomiting, nausea

Gardenia and Soja Combination *(Chih-tzu-shih-tang)*
weak conformation, jaundice, nausea, vomiting, thirst, annoying fever in the chest, insomnia, abdominal distention, thoraco-costal distress, no oliguria

KERATOSIS OF THE PALM

Tang-kuei and Evodia Combination *(Wen-ching-tang)* or
Tang-kuei and Peony Formula *(Tang-kuei-shao-yao-san)*
chills, weak constitution, fever in the palms, dry mouth and lips, abnormal menstruation

Alternate Formulas:

Cinnamon and Hoelen Formula *(Kuei-chih-fu-ling-wan)*
for women of average build with menoxenia and blood stagnancy. More effective if coix is added.

Bupleurum and Peony Formula *(Chia-wei-hsiao-yao-san)*
anorexia, neurosis

Tang-kuei, Evodia, and Ginger Combination *(Tang-kuei-szu-ni-chia-wu-chu-yu-sheng-chiang-tang)*
severe chills, frigorism

Bupleurum and Schizonepeta Combination *(Shih-wei-pai-tu-tang)*
suppuration, felon

KIDNEY PROBLEMS

Formula of Choice:

Hoelen Five Herb Formula *(Wu-ling-san)*
thirst, belching, oliguria, edema

KIDNEY PROBLEMS (Second Stage)

Formula of Choice:

Bupleurum and Hoelen Combination *(Chai-ling-tang)* or Minor Bupleurum Combination with Hoelen Five Herb Formula
belching, anorexia, a dry throat, oliguria, acute gastroenteritis, watery diarrhea, sunstroke, edema, liver disease, cirrhosis, chronic nephritis

Alternate Formulas:

Capillaris and Hoelen Formula *(Yin-chen-wu-ling-san)* or Capillaris Combination with Hoelen Five Herb Formula

a dry mouth, oliguria, vomiting, hangover, edema, jaundice, nephritis

Polyporus Combination *(Chu-ling-tang)*

cystourethritis, oliguria, difficult excretion, increased protein and erythrocyte levels in urine or painful urination, a sensation of residual urine, hematuria

Tang-kuei and Peony Formula *(Tang-kuei-shao-yao-san)*

edema and proteinuria in pregnant women or people with a tendency towards anemia

Rehmannia Eight Formula *(Pa-wei-ti-huang-wan)*

renal atrophy, geriatric nephritis, edema, tinnitus, hypertension, difficult or frequent urination, a dry mouth, lower back pain, lassitude, complications of diabetes mellitus and prostatomegaly

Hoelen and Alisma Combination *(Fen-hsiao-tang* or *Shih-pi-yin)*

ascites, hardening and distention of the abdomen, swelling, oliguria, edema

Gentiana Combination *(Lung-tan-hsieh-kan-tang)*

inflammation of the bladder, urethra, and pudendum; suppuration; for strong people with painful urination due to muscular distention of lower abdomen, a sensation of residual urine, turbid urine and stuttering urination, and in women, leukorrhea

LEUKORRHEA

Formula of Choice:

Lotus Seed Combination *(Ching-hsin-lien-tzu-yin)*
general fatigability, thirst, a dry tongue, oliguria, leukorrhea

Alternate Formulas:

Cinnamon and Dragon Bone Combination *(Kuei-chih-chia-lung-ku-mu-li-tang)*
"flushing up," tendency towards vertigo, chills in the lower body, leukorrhea

Gentiana Combination *(Lung-tan-hsieh-kan-tang)*
for women of average physical strength with inflammation of the vulva, cystitis, and urethritis; leukorrhea

Tang-kuei and Peony Formula *(Tang-kuei-shao-yao-san)*
weak constitution, chills, a tendency towards anemia

Bupleurum and Peony Formula *(Chia-wei-hsiao-yao-san)*
for women of somewhat poor physical strength with anxiety and white or watery leukorrhea

Tang-kuei and Eight Herb Formula *(Pa-wei-tai-hsia-fang)*
for women of less physical strength than that of the Gentiana Combination *(Lung-tan-hsieh-kan-tang)* conformation with a tendency towards anemia and chronic leukorrhea

Rehmannia Eight Formula *(Pa-wei-ti-huang-wan)*
leukorrhea due to geriatric vaginitis

MASTITIS

Formula of Choice:

Pueraria Combination *(Ko-ken-tang)*

pain in a breast from swelling with fear of chills, fever, shoulder stiffness; more effective if combined with platycodon and gypsum

Alternate Formulas:

Bupleurum and Schizonepeta Formula *(Shih-wei-pai-tu-san)*

suppurative mastitis

Platycodon and *Chih-shih* Formula *(Pai-nung-san)*

suppuration, reddening, distention with swelling and hardening

Minor Bupleurum Combination *(Hsiao-chai-hu-tang)*

mastitis, anorexia after a fever has gone

LUMBAGO (Lower Back Pain)

Formula of Choice:

Pueraria Combination *(Ko-ken-tang)*

lower back pain during the initial stage of a common cold or fever

Alternate Formulas:

Rehmannia Eight Formula *(Pa-wei-ti-huang-wan)*

geriatric lumbago, lumbago due to diabetes mellitus, kidney diseases

Tang-kuei and Peony Formula *(Tang-kuei-shao-yao-san)*

lower back pain during pregnancy or after childbirth

Cinnamon and Hoelen Formula *(Kuei-chih-fu-ling-wan)*
abdominal pain and lumbago due to kidney stones, ovaritis, or salpingitis

Persica and Rhubarb Combination *(Tao-ho-cheng-chi-tang)*
lower back pain from a contusion

Tang-kuei*, Cinnamon, and Peony Combination *(Tang-kuei-chien-chung-tang)
chills with pain in the lower abdomen and back

Tang-kuei and Magnolia Formula *(Wu-chi-san)*
lower back pain from chills in the lower body

MENOXENIA, LEUKORRHEA, MENOPAUSAL DISORDERS

Formula of Choice:

Cinnamon and Hoelen Formula *(Kuei-chih-fu-ling-wan)*
for women of average physical strength with pain in the lower abdomen, shoulder stiffness, heavy headedness, vertigo, "flushing up," and cold feet due to menoxenia; menstrual abnormalities, menorrhalgia; menopausal disorders; blood disease

Alternate Formulas:

Bupleurum and Peony Formula *(Chia-wei-hsiao-yao-san)*
for women of weak constitution with shoulder stiffness, fatigability, mental instability, constipation, chills, menoxenia, difficult menstruation, menopausal disorders, and/or blood disease

Tang-kuei and Peony Formula *(Tang-kuei-shao-yao-san)*
for women of little physical strength with chills, a tendency towards anemia, fatigability, occasional pain in the lower abdomen, heavy headedness, vertigo, dizziness, tinnitus, palpitations, shoulder pain, untoned muscles, menoxenia with frequent urination, menstrual abnormalities, menorrhalgia, menopausal disorders

Persica and Rhubarb Combination *(Tao-ho-cheng-chi-tang)*
for women of average physical strength with "flushing up," a tendency towards constipation, headaches, dizziness, vertigo, a cold lower abdomen, menoxenia with lower back pain, difficult menstruation (abdominal pain and severe lower back pain), and mental instability during menstruation and following childbirth

Tang-keui and Gelatin Combination *(Chiung-kuei-chiao-ai-tang)*
anemia due to profuse and prolonged menstruation

Tang-kuei and Evodia Combination *(Wen-ching-tang)*
menoxenia during menopause, prolonged (up to two weeks) and scanty menstruation, fever in the hands and feet, dry mouth and lips, menoxenia, dysmenorrhea, leukorrhea, insomnia, cold feet and loins

Ginseng and Longan Combination *(Kuei-pi-tang)*
weak constitution, anemia due to "flushing up,"

menoxenia, dysmenorrhea, menopausal disorders, neurosis, anxiety

Tang-kuei Four Combination *(Szu-wu-tang)*
dry skin, poor complexion, no gastrointestinal disorders, menoxenia, chills, anemia; aids recovery after childbirth or abortion. Not to be given in presence of gastrointestinal disorders.

Peony and Licorice Combination *(Shao-yao-kan-tsao-tang)*
menorrhalgia, severe pain due to dysmenorrhea

MENTAL PROBLEMS (Instability, Excitability, Mania, Melancholy)

Formula of Choice:

Pinellia and Magnolia Combination *(Pan-hsia-hou-pu-tang)*
vertigo, cardiac hyperfunction, instability, melancholy

Alternate Formulas:

Bupleurum and Peony Formula *(Chia-wei-hsiao-yao-san)*
for women with shoulder stiffness, vertigo, cold feet, "flushing up," and menoxenia due to occluded blood

Ginseng and Longan Combination *(Kuei-pi-tang)*
geriatric neurosis and senility

Bupleurum and Dragon Bone Combination *(Chai-hu-chia-lung-ku-mu-li-tang)*
nervousness, vertigo, palpitations, shoulder stiffness, insomnia

Coptis and Rhubarb Combination *(San-huang-hsieh-hsin-tang)*
for people of medium build with "flushing up," irascibility, excitability, mental instability, constipation

Persica and Rhubarb Combination *(Tao-ho-cheng-chi-tang)*
irascibility at onset of menstruation, mania

Bupleurum Formula *(I-kan-san)*
nervous excitability, irascibility, especially in children

NASAL SUPPURATION, RHINITIS, STUFFY NOSE

Formula of Choice:

Pueraria and Magnolia Flower Combination *(Ko-ken-tang-chia-chiun-chung-hsin-i)*
nasal obstruction, suppurative nasal discharge, distortion of sense of smell, headaches, loss of memory

Alternate Formulas:

Minor Blue Dragon Combination *(Hsiao-ching-lung-tang)*
sensitive rhinitis, nasal discharge

Pueraria Nasal Combination *(Ching-pi-tang)*
for strong people with nasal suppuration, chronic

rhinitis, nasal blockage, heavy headedness, mental instability, and discharge of fetid pus

Magnolia and Gypsum Combination *(Hsin-i-ching-fei-tang)*, Magnolia Flower Formula *(Hsin-i-san)* or Xanthium Formula *(Tsang-erh-san)*

nasal discharge with pus, a feverish sensation and pain in the nose, nasal suppuration, nasal polyps, hypertrophic rhinitis, chronic rhinitis, obstructed breathing, nasal obstruction

Pinellia and Gastrodia Combination *(Pan-hsia-pai-chu-tien-ma-tang)*

weak constitution, poor gastrointestinal tract, cold legs and feet, vertigo, headaches

Bupleurum and Schizonepeta Combination *(Shih-wei-pai-tu-tang)* or Schizonepeta and Forsythia Combination *(Ching-chieh-lien-chiao-tang)*

chronic copius pus with a fetid odor

NEURALGIA, ARTHRITIS (Rheumatalgia)

Formula of Choice:

Coix Combination *(I-yi-jen-tang)*

acute or subacute chronic rheumatic pain; swelling and fever in an infected part which tends to be chronic; difficulty moving the hands and feet, no chills; rheumatism in the hands and feet, arthralgia, muscle pain, pain, paralysis

Alternate Formulas:

Pueraria Combination *(Ko-ken-tang)*

the initial stage of neuralgia, chronic rheumatic pain, sore shoulders, facial neuralgia

Ma-huang and Coix Combination *(Ma-hsin-i-kan-tang)*
usually for chronic rheumatic pain; neuralgia, muscle pain

Cinnamon and Atractylodes Combination *(Kuei-chih-chia-ling-chu-fu-tang)*
for people of little physical strength and a chillphobic constitution with no serious muscular distention, fear of chills, a tendency to perspire, oliguria or frequent urination, painful swelling of the joints in the limbs, difficulty moving, joint pain, neuralgia, pain in the upper body (shoulders, upper arms)

Rehmannia Eight Formula *(Pa-wei-ti-huang-wan)*
cold arms and legs in the elderly, fatigability, oliguria or polyuria, thirst, paralysis, edema; especially for pain in the lower limbs and lower back

Clematis and Stephania Combination *(Shu-ching-huo-hsieh-tang)*
chronic disease with occluded blood, pain in the arms and legs, joint pain, neuralgia, lower back pain, muscle pain; especially for sciatica and pain in the legs

Ophiopogon and Asarum Combination *(Ching-shang-chuan-tung-tang)*
facial pain, headaches, trifacial neuralgia

Tang-kuei and Anemarrhena Combination *(Tang-kuei-nien-tung-tang)*

reddening, swelling, and pain of the muscles around the joints

Persica and Rhubarb Combination *(Tao-ho-cheng-chi-tang)*

for people whose normal complexion is dark and reddish with headaches, constipation, menoxenia, and sciatica

Tu-huo and Vaeicum Combination *(Tu-huo-chi-sheng-tang)*

pain in the loins and knees, chills, numbness, weakness, dysbasia, neuralgia

Peony and Licorice Combination *(Shao-yao-kan-tsao-tang)*

severe pain due to acute muscular spasms, pain in the arms and legs, spasms in the hands and feet

Clematis and Carthamus Formula *(Shu-ching-li-an-san)*

chronic multiple joint pain, pain in the arm and leg joints, neuralgia

NEUROSIS, ANXIETY, INSOMNIA

Formula of Choice:

Ginseng and Longan Combination *(Kuei-pi-tang)* or Ginseng, Bupleurum, and Longan Combination *(Chia-wei-kuei-pi-tang)*

a poor complexion, "flushing up," anemia, amnesia,

palpitations, insomnia due to nervousness and instability

Alternate Formulas:

Pinella and Magnolia Combination *(Pan-hsia-hou-pu-tang)*

melancholy, a sensation of obstruction in the throat

Atractylodes and Hoelen Combination *(Ling-kuei-chu-kan-tang)*

vertigo, dizziness, tinnitus, palpitations, motion sickness

Bupleurum and Dragon Bone Combination *(Chai-hu-chia-lung-ku-mu-li-tang)*

nervousness, mental instability, insomnia, irritation, cardiac hyperfunction, restlessness

Bupleurum and Peony Combination *(Chia-wei-hsiao-yao-san)*

agitation, abdominal swelling, insomnia

Bupleurum and Cinnamon Combination *(Chai-hu-kuei-chih-tang)*

autonomic nerve disorders

Coptis and Scute Combination *(Huang-lien-chieh-tu-tang)* or Coptis and Rhubarb Combination *(San-huang-hsieh-hsin-tang)*

insomnia, insomnia due to hypertension and menopausal disorders. For constipation, Coptis and Rhubarb Combination is advised.

Lotus Seed Combination *(Ching-hsin-lien-tzu-yin)*
weak constitution, involuntary emissions, oliguria, urethral discomfort, insomnia, dry mouth and lips, general fatigue

Minor Cinnamon and Peony Combination *(Hsiao-chien-chung-tang)* or Bupleurum Formula *(I-kan-san)*
children's night terror, night crying

Citrus and Bamboo Combination *(Wen-tan-tang)*
insomnia, irritation, cardiac hyperfunction, terror, nightmares, insomnia due to gastric weakness, neurosis

Zizyphus Combination *(Suan-tsao-jen-tang)*
stress, mental and physical fatigue, irritation, insomnia

Ginseng and Zizyphus Formula *(Tien-wang-pu-hsin-tan)*
insufficient cardiac blood, irritation and excessive sweating, mental instability, constipation, amnesia; also for young people's stress and anxiety

OBESITY

Formula of Choice:

Siler and Platycodon Formula *(Fang-feng-tung-sheng-san)*
firm conformation, obese build, constipation due to lipidosis; for people with a fondness for meat

Alternate Formulas:

Stephania and Astragalus Combination *(Fang-chi-huang-chi-tang)* weak conformation, soft muscles, white skin, obese constitution, fatigability, excessive perspiration, cardiac weakness, edema; mainly the conformation appears in women

Major Bupleurum Combination *(Ta-chai-hu-tang)*
hypertension, distention and hardening beneath the heart, thoraco-costal distress, constipation

Persica and Rhubarb Combination *(Tao-ho-cheng-chi-tang)*
for women of average physical strength with "flushing up," severe vertigo, constipation

OTITIS MEDIA, TINNITUS, HARD OF HEARING, SENSATION OF BLOCKED EAR

Formula of Choice:
Pueraria Combination *(Ko-ken-tang)*
for people of average physical strength; the initial stage of otitis media with fever; fear of chills

Alternate Formulas:
Minor Bupleurum Combination *(Hsiao-chai-hu-tang)*
chronic otitis media, a bitter taste in the mouth, white tongue fur, sore ears, impaired hearing

Bupleurum and Schizonepeta Combination *(Shih-wei-pai-tu-tang)*
suppurative otitis media, otitis externa

Tang-kuei and Astragalus Combination *(Kuei-chi-chien-chung-tang)*

for children and weak people with chronic otitis media that ceaselessly suppurates

Coptis and Rhubarb Combination *(San-huang-hsieh-hsin-tang)*

tinnitus due to hypertension, apoplexy, menopausal disorders

Siler and Platycodon Formula *(Fang-feng-tung-sheng-san)* or Major Bupleurum Combination *(Ta-chai-hu-tang)*

"flushing up," shoulder stiffness, headaches, heavy headedness, thoraco-costal distress, constipation, tinnitus due to obesity, arteriosclerosis, hypertension

Rehmannia Eight Formula *(Pa-wei-ti-huang-wan)* or Scute and Rehmannia Combination *(Tzu-shen-tung-erh-tang)*

for elderly men with tinnitus; impaired hearing; nervous impaired hearing owing to hypofunction of the urological and reproductive organs

Gleditsia Combination *(Tuo-li-hsiao-tu-yin)*

chronic ear problems, incessant suppuration, general weakness, fatigability

PARALYSIS, SPASMS

Formula of Choice:

Pueraria Combination *(Ko-ken-tang)*

for people of average constitution with facial paralysis

Alternate Formulas:

Cinnamon and Atractylodes Combination *(Kuei-chih-chia-ling-chu-fu-tang)*
anxiety, paralysis due to a chillphobic constitution

Rehmannia Eight Formula *(Pa-wei-ti-huang-wan)*
sensory paralysis, numbness, weakness of the legs and feet, dysbasia

Bupleurum and Cinnamon Combination *(Chai-hu-kuei-chih-tang)*
epileptic seizures

Bupleurum and Dragon Bone Combination *(Chai-hu-chia-lung-ku-mu-li-tang)*
nervousness, insomnia, vertigo, palpitations

Coptis and Rhubarb Combination *(San-huang-hsieh-hsin-tang)*
a red complexion, "fire agitation," irascibility, "flushing up"; recommended for prevention of apoplexy

Ma-huang and Ginseng Combination *(Hsu-ming-tang)*
apoplexy, cerebromalacia, hemiplegia, loss of voice

Licorice and Jujube Combination *(Kan-mai-ta-tsao-tang)*
chorea, spasms in women due to hysteria

Bupleurum Formula *(I-kan-san)*
apoplexy, hand tremors due to lesions caused by meningitis. For Parkinson's disease, peony and licorice are usually added.

PEDIATRIC AUTOINTOXICATION

Formula of Choice:

Hoelen Five Herb Formula *(Wu-ling-san)*

thirst, oliguria, nausea, abdominal pain, edema

Alternate Formula:

Ginseng and Ginger Combination *(Jen-sheng-tang)*

cold hands and feet, polyuria, gastric weakness, gastrointestinal weakness, diarrhea, vomiting, stomachache

PEDIATRIC NEUROSIS, NIGHT CRYING, NIGHT TERROR, ENURESIS

Formula of Choice:

Minor Cinnamon and Peony Combination *(Hsiao-chien-chung-tang)*

weak constitution, abdominal flaccidity, fatigability, "flushing up," abdominal pain, palpitations, a feverish feeling in the hands and feet, chills, frequent urination or polyuria

Alternate Formulas:

Licorice and Jujube Combination *(Kan-mai-ta-tsao-tang)*

for children with anxiety, excitability with night crying, night terror, or spasms

Minor Bupleurum Combination *(Hsiao-chai-hu-tang)*

childhood fever or apparent tonsillitis, red and swollen throat, bronchitis, otitis media

Cinnamon and Peony Combination *(Kuei-chih-chia-shao-yao-tang)*
children's night crying with abdominal distention and pain

PSEUDOMYOPIA

Formula of Choice:

Atractylodes and Hoelen Combination *(Ling-kuei-chu-kan-tang)*
dizziness upon standing, heavy headedness, palpitations

Alternate Formula:

Hoelen Five Herb Formula *(Wu-ling-san)*
thirst, oliguria

PULMONARY TUBERCULOSIS AND PLEURITIS

Formula of Choice:

Ginseng and Astragalus Combination *(Pu-chung-i-chi-tang)*
a weak constitution, a weak gastrointestinal tract, fatigability, weakness during convalescence, anorexia, night sweats

Alternate Formulas:

Minor Bupleurum Combination *(Hsiao-chai-hu-tang)* or Bupleurum and Cinnamon Combination *(Chai-hu-kuei-chih-tang)*
anorexia, mild fever, coughing, fatigability, chest pain

Ophiopogon Combination *(Mai-men-tung-tang)*
thick sputum, ceaseless sputum

Scute and Coptis Combination *(Huang-lien-chieh-tu-tang)*
sudden spitting of blood

Phellodendron Combination
(Tzu-yin-chiang-huo-tang)
dark skin, dry sputum difficult to expectorate, hemoptysis, dry throat, severe cough with ceaseless sputum

PYORRHEA ALVEOLARIS

Formula of Choice:

Pueraria Combination *(Ko-ken-tang)*
the initial stage of painful gingival swelling

Alternate Formulas:

Platycodon and *Chih-shih* Formula *(Pai-nung-san)*
suppurative diseases

Cinnamon Five Herb Combination *(Kuei-chih-wu-wu-tang)*
gingivitis, tooth decay, pyorrhea alveolaris, gingival swelling and reddening; for constipation add rhubarb; for inflammation add gypsum

Coptis and Rehmannia Combination *(Ching-wei-san)*
fever in the stomach or mouth, halitosis, tongue fur, toothache, gingival ulcers, gingival pain, hemorrhage

REDUCED SEXUAL DESIRE

Formula of Choice:

Lycium Formula *(Huan-shao-tan)*

insufficient sperm, loss of appetite, weakness not due to age, reduced sexual desire, anorexia, fever and night sweats, mental weakness, lower back pain, lassitude; also warms the uterus, improves the skin

Alternate Formulas:

Cinnamon and Dragon Bone Combination *(Kuei-chih-chia-lung-ku-mu-li-tang)*

a weak constitution, fatigability, excitability, nervousness, insomnia, night crying, bedwetting, eye fatigue, impotence, nervous cardiac palpitations

Bupleurum and Dragon Bone Combination *(Chai-hu-chia-lung-ku-mu-li-tang)*

Cinnamon and Dragon Bone Combination symptoms with mental instability, severe nervousness, palpitations, insomnia; climacteric neurosis

Rehmannia Six Formula *(Liu-wei-ti-huang-wan)*

a tonic for the kidneys; used for weakness in the loins and knees, vertigo, tinnitus, deafness, emissions, cold arms and legs, fatigability

Rehmannia Eight Formula *(Pa-wei-ti-huang-wan)*

a tonic that warms the kidneys; used for chills and pain in the loins and knees, oliguria, incontinence, polyuria, thirst, edema, diarrhea, impotence

Ginseng and *Tang-kuei* Ten Combination *(Shih-chuan-ta-pu-tang)*

a tonic for the elderly; used for insufficiency of blood, amnesia, anemia, cold hands and feet, lassitude, anorexia, baldness. More effective if cervus is added.

Lotus Stamen Formula *(Chin-suo-ki-ching-wan)*

for young men with involuntary emissions, lower back pain, tinnitus, and weak arms and legs

SHOULDER STIFFNESS

Formula of Choice:

Pueraria Combination *(Ko-ken-tang)*

pain in the neck and back

Alternate Formulas:

Major Bupleurum Combination *(Ta-chai-hu-tang)*

for muscular people with obstinate shoulder stiffness and constipation

Minor Bupleurum Combination *(Hsiao-chai-hu-tang)*

for people of normal or somewhat weak physical strength and an adenosis constitution with a bitter mouth at rising, a dry mouth, thoraco-costal distress, a sensation of pressure, and shoulder stiffness

Bupleurum and Dragon Bone Combination *(Chai-hu-chia-lung-ku-mu-li-tang)*

cardiac hyperfunction, insomnia, vertigo, constipation, shoulder stiffness with excitability

Bupleurum and Peony Formula *(Chia-wei-hsiao-yao-san)*
shoulder stiffness with menoxenia and leukorrhea

Tang-kuei and Peony Formula *(Tang-kuei-shao-yao-san)*
for women with shoulder stiffness, weakness, chills, menoxenia

Cinnamon and Hoelen Formula *(Kuei-chih-fu-ling-wan)*
headaches and shoulder stiffness due to occluded blood. If the person has a muscular constitution with constipation, Persica and Rhubarb Combination *(Tao-ho-cheng-chi-tang)* is used instead.

Evodia Combination *(Wu-chu-yu-tang)*
a stiff neck, severe paroxysmal headaches, shoulder stiffness

Pinellia Combination *(Pan-hsia-hsieh-hsin-tang)* or Six Major Herb Combination *(Liu-chun-tzu-tang)*
shoulder stiffness with gastric weakness

STOMATITIS

Formula of Choice:

Sweet Combination *(Kan-lu-yin)*
erosion and suppuration of the mouth, tongue, gingiva, throat due to stagnant fever in the digestive system

Alternate Formulas:

Tang-kuei and Gardenia Combination *(Wen-ching-yin)*
poor complexion, "flushing up," climacteric disorders,

neurosis, menoxenia, difficult menstruation, dermatitis, hemorrhage

Coptis and Scute Combination *(Huang-lien-chieh-tu-tang)*
for strong people with "flushing up," facial reddening, and stomatitis with mental instability

Capillaris Combination *(Yin-chen-hao-tang)*
thirst, oliguria, hives with constipation, stomatitis

STOMATOCACE (Ulcerative Stomatitis)

Formula of Choice:

Sweet Combination *(Kan-lu-yin)*
gingivitis, halitosis, ulcerative stomatitis, painful swelling in the throat

SUPPURATION

Formula of Choice:

Bupleurum and Schizonepeta Formula *(Shih-wei-pai-tu-tang)*
the initial stage of mild suppurative skin diseases such as pimples, boils, carbuncles, lymphnoditis, felon

Alternate Formulas:

Schizonepeta and Siler Formula *(Ching-fang-pai-tu-san)*
the initial stage of acute suppuration with fever, headaches, reddening, swelling, and pain

Coptis and Scute Combination *(Huang-lien-chieh-tu-tang)*
"flushing up," occluded blood, hemorrhage

Gleditsia Combination *(Tuo-li-hsiao-tu-yin)*
for people of somewhat weak conformation with suppurative disease, glandular inflammation, a multiple muscle inflammation; speeds suppuration and releases poison in the body

Tang-kuei, Astragalus, and Peony Combination *(Kuei-chi-chien-chung-tang)*
for people weaker than the Gleditsia Combination conformation with chronic ulcers and suppurative swelling

TONSILLITIS, HYPERTROPHY, PAIN IN THE LARYNX

Formula of Choice:

Pueraria Combination *(Ko-ken-tang)*
the initial stage of the disease—excessive sweating, fear of chills, headaches, fever; for severe sore throat add platycodon and gypsum

Alternate Formulas:

Minor Bupleurum Combination *(Hsiao-chai-hu-tang)*
fever lasting two to three weeks, white tongue fur, mild fever, thoraco-costal distress

Gardenia and Mentha Combination *(Ching-liang-yin)*
severe sore throat lasting three to four days with inflammation, occluded blood

Bupleurum and Pueraria Combination *(Chai-ko-chieh-chi-tang)* good for a sore and swollen throat with fever

Bupleurum and Rehmannia Combination *(Chai-hu-ching-kan-tang)*
children's adenosis constitution; tonsillar hypertrophy, severe cough, sore throat

Platycodon Combination *(Chieh-keng-tang)*
swollen throat, pain with suppuration, peritonsillitis

URTICARIA, ECZEMA

Formula of Choice:

Bupleurum and Schizonepeta Formula *(Shih-wei-pai-tu-tang)*
the initial stage of suppurative skin diseases and acute skin diseases; urticaria, acute eczema, athlete's foot, carbuncles, pimples

Alternate Formulas:

Pueraria Combination *(Ko-ken-tang)*
the initial stage of urticaria with swelling, reddening, itching, fear of chills, and fever. For constipation, add rhubarb. For severe itching, add gypsum.

Tang-kuei and Arctium Formula *(Hsiao-feng-san)*
obstinate chronic eczema with suppuration, scabbing, itching, thirst

Tang-kuei and Gardenia Combination *(Wen-ching-yin)*
dry skin with a burning sensation, poor complexion, "flushing up," severe itching when warm. A combin-

ation of *Tang-kuei* Four Combination *(Szu- wu-tang)* and Coptis and Scute Combination *(Huang- lien-chieh- tu-tang)* is effective for occluded blood and inflammation; it induces tranquility.

Minor Bupleurum Combination *(Hsiao-chai-hu-tang)* or Major Bupleurum Combination *(Ta-chai-hu-tang)*
chronic eczema due to liver disorders; for people prone to skin or suppurative diseases

Bupleurum and Peony Formula *(Chia-wei-hsiao-yao-san)*
chronic urticaria; women's diseases such as menoxenia

Rehmannia Eight Formula *(Pa-wei-ti-huang-wan)*
geriatric itching

Ludwigia Formula *(Teng-hua-pai-tu-san)*
the initial stage of urticaria. An antidote for poison, it relieves inflammation and smooths urination.

Ginseng and Mentha Formula *(Jen-sheng-pai-tu-san)*
for people of weak constitution

VAGINITIS, VAGINAL ECZEMA, ITCHING AND PAIN, ENDOMETRITIS

Formula of Choice:

Gentiana Combination *(Lung-tan-hsieh-kan-tang)*
for people of average physical strength with a tendency towards muscular distention in the lower abdomen; vaginitis, vaginal eczema, leukorrhea,

vaginal itching and pain, endometritis, painful urination, a sensation of residual urine, turbid urine

Alternate Formulas:

Tang-kuei and Peony Formula *(Tang-kuei-shao-yao-san)*
physical weakness, anemia, chills

Tang-kuei Eight Herb Formula *(Pa-wei-tai-hsia-fang)*
weak constitution, anemia, gonococcal leukorrhea, chronic diseases

VERTIGO

Formula of Choice:

Atractylodes and Hoelen Combination *(Ling-kuei-chu-kan-tang)*
vertigo upon standing, Meniere's disease

Alternate Formulas:

Pinellia and Magnolia Combination *(Pan-hsia-hou-pu-tang)*
mild vertigo or a sensation of instability

Pinellia and Gastrodia Combination *(Pan-hsia-pai-chu-tien-ma-tang)*
vertigo due to gastroptosis or gastric weakness with headaches

Tang-kuei and Peony Formula *(Tang-kuei-shao-yao-san)*
menopausal disorders, vertigo due to childbirth

Coptis and Rhubarb Combination *(San-huang-hsieh-hsin-tang)* or Coptis and Scute Combination *(Huang-lien-chieh-tu-tang)*

hypertension, red complexion, "flushing up"

Vitality Combination *(Chen-wu-tang)*

vertigo due to hypotension, general weakness, cold hands and feet, fatigability

VOMITING OF PREGNANCY

Formula of Choice:

Minor Pinellia and Hoelen Combination *(Hsiao-pan-hsia-chia-fu-ling-tang)*

for pregnant women in the first months with vomiting and nausea, distention and fullness below the sternum, stagnant water beneath the heart, vertigo, palpitations, and thirst

Alternate Formulas:

Hoelen Five Herb Formula *(Wu-ling-san)*

thirst, oliguria; used with Minor Pinellia and Hoelen Combination *(Hsiao-pan-hsia-chia-fu-ling-tang)*

Pinellia and Magnolia Combination *(Pan-hsia-hou-pu-tang)*

mental instability, a sensation of distention and fullness from the throat to the chest, stomach distention with nausea and vomiting

Pinellia Combination *(Pan-hsia-hsieh-hsin-tang)*
stomach distention, nausea, anorexia

Evodia Combination *(Wu-chu-yu-tang)*
severe headaches with vomiting and stagnant water

IV. FORMULAS AND SYMPTOMS

(The symbol ★ means that a herbal formula has been approved for use in medical facilities by the Department of Pharmaceutical Affairs, Ministry of Health and Welfare, Japan.)

(The symbol ☆ means that a herbal formula has been approved for use in medical facilities by the National Health Administration, Republic of China.)

The book title under the formula name is that of the original source of the formula.

☆ ★ Apricot Seed and Linum Formula *(Ma-tzu-jen-wan)* 麻子仁丸

Shang han lun, Chin kuei yao lueh

Herbs: linum, peony, *chih-shih*, magnolia, apricot seed, rhubarb.

Uses: a mild cathartic; for elderly people with general weakness or constipation during convalescence, habitual constipation (weakness), or hemorrhoids due to constipation

★ **Areca and Evodia Combination** ***(Pien-chih-hsin-chi-yin)*** 變製心氣飲
Japanese formula

Herbs: cinnamon, areca seed, hoelen, pinellia, akebia, perilla fruit, tortoise shell, *chih-shih,* morus, licorice, evodia

Uses: palpitations, gasping, edema, shoulder and back stiffness; cardiac asthma; chronic bronchitis; angina pectoris

☆ **Areca Seed Combination** ***(Chiu-ping-wu-fu-tang)*** 九檳吳茯湯
Chang tsang yen fang

Herbs: areca seed, magnolia, cinnamon bark, citrus, ginger, akebia, perilla, licorice, evodia, hoelen, rhubarb

Uses: beriberi, swelling due to beriberi, gasping, general lassitude

★ **Astragalus Combination** ***(Huang-chi-chien-chung-tang)*** 黄耆建中湯
Chin kuei yao lueh

Herbs: peony, cinnamon, ginger, jujube, licorice, astragalus, maltose

Uses: for people of chronic weak constitution suffering from suppurative disease and overwork, or not recovering from an illness; weakness during convalescence; a weak constitution; excessive sweating; night sweats; otitis media; chronic ulcers; anal fistula; debilitation in children; and carbuncles and furunculosis

★ Astragalus and Atractylodes Combination *(Ching-shu-i-chi-tang)* 清暑益氣湯

I hsueh liu yao

Herbs: ginseng, atractylodes, ophiopogon, *tang-kuei*, astragalus, citrus, schizandra, phellodendron, licorice, alisma, *shen-chu*, blue citrus peel

Effects: an altered form of Ginseng and Astragalus Combination *(Pu-chung-i-chi-tang)*; strengthens *ch'i*, dissipates fever

Uses: illness due to summer heat, excessive sweating, thirst, annoying fever, yellowish red urine, sunstroke, irradiation sickness, anorexia due to hot weather, diarrhea, general lassitude, emaciation in the summer

★ Astragalus and Platycodon Formula *(Chien-chin-nei-tuo-san)* 千金内托散

Wan ping hui chun

Herbs: ginseng, *tang-kuei*, astragalus, cnidium, siler, platycodon, magnolia, cinnamon, angelica, licorice

Effects: improves the recovery mechanism

Uses: suppurative diseases, weakness, a tendency towards exhaustion, carbuncles, facial boils, suppurative mastitis, suppurative otitis media, otorrhea, suppurating lungs, periproctitis, anal fistula, skin ulcer, bone necrosis

☆ **Atractylodes Combination** ***(Yueh-pi-chia-chu-tang)*** 越婢加朮湯
Chin kuei yao lueh

Herbs: *ma-huang*, gypsum, atractylodes, ginger, licorice, jujube

Effects: eases urination, eliminates edema and pain

Uses: edema, dermatosis, urological diseases, ophthalmological diseases, acute nephritis, nephritis, rheumatic degenerative arthritis, eczema, acute conjunctivitis

★ **Bamboo and Hoelen Combination** ***(Wen-tan-tang)*** 温膽湯
Chien chin fang

Herbs: pinellia, hoelen, ginger, citrus, bamboo, *chih-shih*, licorice (sometimes with coptis and zizyphus)

Uses: for people of atonic constitution with insomnia due to gastroptosis, gastric atonia, or gastrointestinal weakness; neurosis; palpitations, cardiac hyperfunction; gastrointestinal disorders

Bamboo and Gypsum Combination ***(Chu-yeh-shih-kao-tang)*** 竹葉石膏湯
Shang han lun

Herbs: ophiopogon, oryza, pinellia, ginseng, bamboo, licorice, gypsum

Uses: pneumonia, measles, influenza or febrile diseases, mild fever after a severe fever, cough, thirst, excessive sweating, night sweats, lack of body fluids, dry skin, loss of physical strength, irritation in the chest, gasping, vomiting, white tongue fur; bronchitis, whooping cough, bronchial asthma, pulmonary emphysema, pulmonary tuberculosis, lung abscess, diabetes mellitus; a weak, hollow and frequent pulse

★ **Bupleurum Formula** ***(I-kan-san)*** 抑肝散
Chih chih fang

Herbs: *tang-kuei*, gambir, cnidium, atractylodes, hoelen, bupleurum, licorice

Effects: arrests liver illnesses

Uses: disturbance of *ch'i* in the liver, weak constitution, neurosis, irascibility, excitability, insomnia, nervousness, epilepsy, hysteria, night crying in children, neurotic wryneck

★ **Bupleurum and Cinnamon Combination *(Chai-hu-kuei-chih-tang)*** 柴胡桂枝湯
Shang han lun, Chin kuei yao lueh

Herbs: scute, bupleurum, pinellia, cinnamon, ginseng, peony, ginger, jujube, licorice. Combines Minor Bupleurum Combination *(Hsiao-chai-hu-tang)* and Cinnamon Combination *(Kuei-chih-tang)*

Uses: prolonged and exacerbated common cold, persistent fever, tension in the chest and abdomen, weak gastrointestinal tract, gastritis, mild fever, fear of chills, headaches, common cold with nausea, cholelithiasis with severe pain, anorexia, pleuritis, severe pain in the stomach and abdomen

★ **Bupleurum, Cinnamon, and Ginger Combination *(Chai-hu-kuei-chih-kan-chiang-tang)*** 柴胡桂枝乾薑湯
Shang han lun

Herbs: bupleurum, cinnamon, trichosanthes root, scute, *oyster shell,* licorice, ginger

Uses: physical and mental weakness, poor complexion, a tendency toward anemia, palpitations, gasping, nervousness, mild fever, cough, insomnia, abnormal heartbeat, diarrhea, common cold, neurasthenia, insomnia, cardiac asthma and palpitations, menopausal disorders, menopausal neurosis, neurosis

★ **Bupleurum and Dragon Bone Combination** ***(Chai-hu-chia-lung-ku-mu-li-tang)*** 柴胡加龍骨牡蠣湯
Shang han lun, Chin kuei yao lueh

Herbs: bupleurum, pinellia, hoelen, cinnamon, scute, jujube, ginger, ginseng, dragon bone, oyster shell, rhubarb

Uses: for adults of average physical strength suffering from mental instability, palpitations, insomnia, constipation, and dizziness; for nervous children or those with symptoms of epilepsy; for arteriosclerosis, hypertension, and complications of hypertension such as palpitations, insomnia, and instability; and for habitual insomnia, nephritis, epilepsy, heart disease, menopausal neurosis, and night crying in children

★ **Bupleurum and Hoelen Combination** ***(Chai-ling-tang)*** 柴苓湯
Te hsiao fang

Herbs: bupleurum, pinellia, scute, ginseng, jujube, ginger, licorice, cinnamon, polyporus, atractylodes, hoelen, alisma. Combines Minor Bupleurum Combination *(Hsiao-chai-hu-tang)* and Hoelen Five Herb Formula *(Wu-ling-san)*.

Uses: thirst, oliguria, edema or diarrhea, common cold, acute gastritis, nephritis, pyelitis

★ **Bupleurum and Peony Formula** ***(Chia-wei-hsiao-yao-san)*** 加味逍遙散
Ho chi chu fang

Herbs: *tang-kuei*, peony, bupleurum, white atractylodes, hoelen, ginger, licorice, mentha, moutan, gardenia

Uses: menopausal disorders, menoxenia, neurosis due to abortion or sterilization, mental instability, fatigability, headaches, shoulder stiffness, constipation, lumbago, dysmenorrhea, menopausal neurosis, hysteria, neurasthenia, insomnia

☆ **Bupleurum and Pueraria Combination** ***(Chai-ko-chieh-chi-tang)*** 柴葛解肌湯
Shang han liu shu

Herbs: bupleurum, pueraria, scute, peony, chianghuo, angelica, platycodon, licorice, jujube, gypsum, dried ginger

Uses: used if *Ma-huang* Combination *(Ma-huang-tang)*, Cinnamon Combination *(Kuei-chih-tang)*, or Pueraria Combination *(Ko-ken-tang)* fail to relieve the fever of a common cold or influenza; also for thirst and annoying pain in the limbs, common cold, pneumonia, febrile diseases

★ **Bupleurum and Scute Combination** ***(Chai-hsien-tang)*** 柴陷湯
Shen shih tsun sheng shu

Herbs: bupleurum, pinellia, scute, ginger, jujube, trichosanthes seed, licorice, ginseng, coptis. Combines Minor Bupleurum Combination *(Hsiao-chai-hu-tang)* and Minor Trichosanthes Combination *(Hsiao-hsien-hsiung-tang).*

Uses: a sensation of fullness and pressure in the chest, chest pain when coughing or breathing deeply, sticky sputum difficult to expectorate, gasping, alternating chills and fever; bronchitis, pneumonia, pleuritis, common cold

★ **Bupleurum and Schizonepeta Combination** ***(Shih-wei-pai-tu-tang)*** 十味敗毒湯
S. Hanaoka

Herbs: bupleurum, cherry bark, platycodon, ginger, cnidium, hoelen, *tu-huo*, siler, licorice, schizonepeta

Effects: adjusts autonomic nervous system and glandular excretions, strengthens the liver, improves resistance in allergic constitutions; an external medication (dressing)

Uses: urticaria, eczema, athlete's foot, pimples, the initial stage of acute skin disease, suppurative skin disease

★ Capillaris Combination *(Yin-chen-hao-tang)*
茵陳蒿湯

Shang han lun, Chin kuei yao lueh

Herbs: capillaris, gardenia, rhubarb

Uses: stagnancy in the chest, a sensation of vomiting, thirst, oliguria even though the patient has drunk water, hepatitis, nephrosclerosis, food poisoning, urticaria, stomatitis, cholecystisis; especially famous for treating jaundice

★ Capillaris and Hoelen Formula *(Yin-chen-wu-ling-san)* 茵陳五苓散

Shang han lun, Chin kuei yao lueh

Herbs: capillaris, alisma, polyporus, atractylodes, cinnamon, hoelen. Hoelen Five Herb Formula plus capillaris.

Uses: thirst, oliguria, liver disorders or a tendency towards jaundice, hepatitis, nephritis, nephrosclerosis, ascites, vomiting, urticaria, vomiting and edema due to hangover

★ Cardamon and Fennel Formula *(An-chung-san)*
安中散

Ho chi chu fang

Herbs: cinnamon, corydalis, oyster shell, fennel, licorice, cardamon, galanga

Uses: fear of chills; anxiety; gastrointestinal pain; upset stomach; weak constitution; emaciation; a tendency towards flaccid abdominal muscles, stomachache or abdominal pain; a burning sensation in the chest; hiccoughs; anorexia; nausea; fondness for sweets; gastrointestinal illness, chronic gastritis, neurotic gastritis, gastrosia, or chronic stomachache. Since the formula does not contain soda, it is good for chronic gastritis and/or intoxication due to long-term use of soda.

☆ **Chrysanthemum Combination *(Tzu-sheng-ming-mu-tang)*** 滋腎明目湯
Wan ping huei chun

Herbs: *tang-kuei*, peony, cnidium, raw rehmannia, cured rehmannia, platycodon, ginseng, gardenia, coptis, angelica, vitex, chrysanthemum, licorice, juncus, tea

Uses: dysopia from weakness due to persistent disease or weak *ch'i* and blood; cataracts; eye fatigability

★ **Cimicifuga Combination *(I-tzu-tang)*** 乙字湯
Yuan nan yang

Herbs: rhubarb, bupleurum, cimicifuga, licorice, scute, *tang-kuei*

Effects: improves hepatic function and blood circulation with continuous use; eliminates constipation. The best formula in Chinese medicine for hemorrhoids.

Uses: hemorrhoids; hemorrhoidal fissures, pain, and bleeding; the initial stage of anal prolapse; constipation; hard stools

★ Cinnamon Combination *(Kuei-chih-tang)* 桂枝湯
Shang han lun

Herbs: cinnamon, peony, jujube, ginger, licorice

Uses: greater yang disease; weak constitution plus external weakness; a floating and weak pulse, fear of chills or wind, fever, headaches, spontaneous sweating; general neurosis; rheumatism; abdominal pain due to chills; neurasthenia; impotence; involuntary emissions

Cinnamon and Anemarrhena Combination *(Kuei-chih-shao-yao-chih-mu-tang)* 桂枝芍藥知母湯
Chin kuei yao lueh

Herbs: cinnamon, anemarrhena, siler, peony, *ma-huang*, ginger, atractylodes, licorice, aconite

Uses: persistent swelling pain in the joints with weak physical strength, chronic arthritis

Cinnamon and Astragalus Combination *(Kuei-chih-chia-huang-chi-tang)* 桂枝加黄耆湯
Chin kuei yao lueh

Herbs: cinnamon, peony, jujube, ginger, astragalus, licorice

Uses: edematous skin, lack of flexibility, night sweats, a sensation of numbness, excessive sweating, otitis media, phlyctenule, skin disease

★ Cinnamon, Atractylodes, and Aconite Combination *(Kuei-chih-chia-chu-fu-tang)* 桂枝加朮附湯
Todo Yoshimasu

Herbs: cinnamon, peony, jujube, ginger, licorice, atractylodes, aconite

Uses: chronic neuralgia, rheumatalgia, soreness and pain due to a common cold, limb paralysis, difficulty bending at the waist, arthritis, paralysis, spasms

★ Cinnamon and Dragon Bone Combination *(Kuei-chih-chia-lung-ku-mu-li-tang)* 桂枝加龍骨牡蠣湯
Shang han lun, Chin kuei yao lueh

Herbs: cinnamon, peony, jujube, ginger, licorice, dragon bone, oyster shell. Cinnamon Combination *(Kuei-chih-tang)* plus dragon bone and oyster shell.

Effects: tranquilizes and strengthens the body

Uses: for weak people with symptoms of excitability and fatigability; neurosis; loss of vitality; impotence; involuntary emissions; infertility; baldness

★ **Cinnamon Five Herb Combination *(Kuei-chih-wu-wu-tang)*** 桂枝五物湯
Todo Yoshimasu

Herbs: cinnamon, scute, rehmannia, hoelen, platycodon

Uses: firm conformation with toothache, gingivitis, erosion of the mouth and tongue, or pyorrhea alveolaris

★ **Cinnamon and Ginseng Combination *(Kuei-chih-jen-sheng-tang)*** 桂枝人參湯
Shang han lun

Herbs: cinnamon, ginseng, atractylodes, licorice, ginger

Uses: surface fever and interior chills, namely, headache, fever, perspiration, fear of chills; stagnancy and hardening beneath the heart; gastrointestinal weakness, diarrhea; pain in the heart and abdomen, palpitations beneath the heart; lassitude in the limbs, chills in the feet; polyuria; chills; gastroenteritis; gastric weakness; colitis; chronic diarrhea; migraine; habitual headaches; palpitations; acute spasms in children; common cold; influenza; a weak conformation

★ **Cinnamon and Hoelen Formula** ***(Kuei-chih-fu-ling-wan)*** 桂枝茯苓丸
Chin kuei yao lueh

Herbs: cinnamon, hoelen, moutan, persica, peony

Effects: similar to *Tang-kuei* and Peony Formula *(Tang-kuei-shao-yao-san)*; improves blood circulation, dispels occluded blood

Uses: for people of relatively average physical strength with disturbances of liver, fear of chilling in the lower body, occasional pain in the lower abdomen, shoulder stiffness, "flushing up," vertigo, heavy headedness, sore shoulders, coarse skin, menoxenia, disorders due to menoxenia or menopause, leukorrhea, menopausal neurosis, eczema, freckles, chronic appendicitis, contusions, frigorism or internal hemorrhaging due to wounds

★ **Cinnamon and Peony Combination** ***(Kuei-chih-chia-shao-yao-tang)*** 桂枝加芍藥湯
Shang han lun

Herbs: cinnamon, peony, jujube, ginger, licorice

Uses: chills, abdominal distention, abdominal pain, occasional diarrhea, colitis, peritonitis, proctitis, hernia

☆ **Clematis and Carthamus Formula** ***(Shu-chin-li-an-san)*** 舒筋立安散
Wan ping huei chun

Herbs: siler, *tu-huo,* cnidium, chianghuo, angelica, hoelen, achyranthes, licorice, rehmannia, atractylodes, peony, carthamus, persica, pinellia, aurantium, chaenomeles, stephania, clematis, forsythia, akebia, gentiana, scute, bamboo sap, processed aconite, citrus, arisaema

Uses: joint pain in the limbs, acute or chronic arthritic rheumatism, hemiplegia. Suitable for long term use.

★ **Clematis and Stephania Combination** ***(Shu-ching-huo-hsieh-tang)*** 疏經活血湯
Wan ping huei chun

Herbs: *tang-kuei*, rehmannia, peony, atractylodes, persica, achyranthes, clematis, citrus, cnidium, chianghuo, siler, angelica, hoelen, gentiana, licorice, stephania, ginger

Uses: physical weakness due to overindulgence in alcohol and sex; lingering pain in the body, especially in the left leg and foot, that becomes more severe at night; neuralgia, sciatica, muscular rheumatism, joint pain, lower back pain

☆★ **Cnidium and Tea Formula** ***(Chuan-chiung-cha-tiao-san)*** 川芎茶調散

Herbs: mentha, cnidium, schizonepeta, chianghuo, angelica, licorice, siler, tea, cyperus

Uses: vertigo, heavy headedness, migraine, common cold, headache, stuffy nose, menopausal neurosis

★ **Coix Combination** ***(I-yi-jen-tang)*** 薏苡仁湯
Ming i chih chang

Herbs: coix, *tang-kuei*, peony, *ma-huang*, cinnamon, atractylodes, licorice

Uses: pain in the limb joints, swelling, a feverish sensation, subacute arthritic rheumatism, muscular rheumatism, arthritis, muscular pain, neuralgia

Coptis and Rehmannia Formula ***(Ching-wei-san)*** 清胃散
I tsung chin chien

Herbs: gypsum, moutan, scute, rehmannia, coptis, cimicifuga

Uses: firm fire in the stomach, hemorrhaging of the gums between the teeth, swelling pain in the gingiva, stomatitis, swelling pain in the throat, toothache

★ Coptis and Rhubarb Combination *(San-huang-hsieh-hsin-tang)* 三黃瀉心湯 or ★ Coptis and Rhubarb Formula *(San-huang-ting)* 三黃錠

Chin kuei yao lueh

Herbs: rhubarb, scute, coptis

Effects: prevents apoplexy

Uses: a red complexion in a person with a constitution susceptible to apoplexy, fire agitation, irascibility, and insomnia; habitual constipation in physically strong people; for people of average physical strength with a tendency to "flush up," a red complexion, mental instability, and a tendency to be constipated; apoplexy; hypertension; insomnia; hemoptysis; nosebleed; metrorrhagia; climacteric disorders; hemorrhoidal bleeding; blood disease; conjunctival congestion and hemorrhage; burns, stomachache

★ Cyperus and Perilla Formula *(Hsiang-su-san)* 香蘇散

Ho chi chu fang

Herbs: cyperus, citrus, ginger, perilla, licorice

Uses: initial stage of mild common cold, stagnancy beneath the heart, depression, gastric weakness, anxiety, common cold with vomiting of gastric acid and belching, neurasthenia, food poisoning

Dandelion Combination *(Pu-kung-ying-tang)* 蒲公英湯
Fang yu ni

Herbs: dandelion, *tang-kuei*, dioscorea, cyperus, moutan

Uses: insufficient milk within one month after childbirth

★ Evodia Combination *(Wu-chu-yu-tang)* 吳茱萸湯
Shang han lun, Chin kuei yao lueh

Herbs: evodia, ginseng, jujube, ginger

Effects: warms the kidneys, removes chills, stops vomiting and diarrhea

Uses: stagnant water in the stomach, distention beneath the heart, chills in the hands and feet, vomiting, headaches, migraine, habitual headaches, nausea with headaches, hiccoughs

★ Four Major Herb Combination *(Szu-chun-tzu-tang)* 四君子湯

Ho chi chu fang

Herbs: ginseng, atractylodes, hoelen, licorice, ginger, jujube

Effects: strengthens the spleen and stomach, improves appetite

Uses: diseases that reduce vitality; emaciation, poor complexion, anorexia, fatigability, gastrointestinal weakness, anemia, gastric weakness, gastroptosis, gastric ulcer, chronic gastritis, a sensation of pressure in the stomach, diarrhea

★ Gambir Formula *(Kou-teng-san)* 鈎藤散

Pen shih fang

Herbs: gambir, citrus, pinellia, ophiopogon, hoelen, ginseng, chrysanthemum, siler, gypsum, ginger, licorice

Uses: for people past middle age with neurosis and/or a tendency towards hypertension; chronic persistent headaches; vertigo; shoulder stiffness; hypertension; headaches due to arteriosclerosis; neurotic headaches; insomnia

★ Gardenia and Mentha Combination *(Ching-liang-yin)* 清涼飲

Wan ping huei chun

Herbs: gardenia, forsythia, scute, siler, *tang-kuei*, rehmannia, licorice, platycodon, *chih-ko*, coptis, mentha, angelica, juncus, tea

Uses: firm fire and swelling pain in the throat, tonsillitis

Gardenia and Soja Combination *(Chih-tzu-shih-tang)* 梔子豉湯

Shang han lun, Chin kuei yao lueh

Herbs: gardenia, soja

Effects: gardenia reduces inflammation and fever and sedates, soja tranquilizes

Uses: weak conformation, stagnant *ch'i* in the chest, annoyance in the heart, melancholy, annoying fever, stagnant pain in the heart, jaundice, esophageal stenosis, insomnia, neurosis, stomatitis, gastritis, esophageal cancer, hemorrhaging, chest pain

☆ Gardenia and Vitex Combination *(Hsi-kan-ming-mu-tang)* 洗肝明目湯

Wan ping huei chun

Herbs: *tang-kuei*, peony, cnidium, rehmannia, scute, gardenia, forsythia, siler, cassia seed, coptis, schizonepeta, mentha, chianghuo, vitex, chrysanthemum, platycodon, tribulus, licorice, gypsum

Uses: eye disease of a firm fever conformation; corneal and conjunctival diseases with inflammation, congestion, and pain; sclerosing keratitis, keratitis, scleritis, iritis

★ Gasping Formula ***(Hsiang-sheng-po-ti-wan)***
響聲破笛丸
Wan ping huei chun

Herbs: forsythia, platycodon, licorice, rhubarb, cardamon, cnidium, terminalia, catechu, mentha

Uses: hoarseness due to excessive talking and singing, general hoarseness, throat pain

Gentiana Combination ***(Lung-tan-hsieh-kan-tang)***
龍膽瀉肝湯
Hsueh shih i an

Herbs: gentiana, bupleurum, alisma, akebia, plantago, rehmannia, *tang-kuei*, gardenia, scute, licorice

Effects: eliminates fever and inflammation, cools and freshens the blood, eases urination, moderates the condition

Uses: people of average physical strength with inflammation in the lower abdomen and pudendum, a tendency towards tension in the lower abdomen, congestion, swelling and pain; cystitis, urethritis, vaginitis, abnormal leukorrhea, endometritis, pudendal pruritis, gonorrhea, vulvitis, and pudendal eczema

Ginseng Combination *(Tu-sheng-tang)* 獨參湯

Herbs: 15-30g of ginseng decocted

Effects: strengthens *ch'i* and the organs

Uses: shock due to severe hemorrhaging, severe diarrhea, and severe vomiting; severe hemorrhaging

Ginseng and Akebia Combination *(Pu-chung-chih-shih-tang)* 補中治溼湯
***I lin chi yao* (Corrections of Medicine)**

Herbs: ginseng, white atractylodes, atractylodes, hoelen, citrus, ophiogpogon, *tang-kuei*, akebia, scute, magnolia, cimicifuga. An altered form of Magnolia and Alisma Combination *(Pu-chi-chien-chung-tang).*

Uses: a weak conformation with distention, ascites, and edema—for edema in a firm conformation, Bupleurum and Hoelen Combination *(Chai-ling-tang)*, Hoelen and Alisma Combination *(Fen-hsiao-tang)*, or Hoelen Five Herb Formula *(Wu-ling-san)* is used; ascites; cirrhosis; chronic peritonitis; chronic nephritis; nephralgia; edema due to valvular disease

★☆ Ginseng and Astragalus Combination *(Pu-chung-i-chi-tang)* 補中益氣湯
Pien huo lun

Herbs: astragalus, ginseng, atractylodes, *tang-kuei*, citrus, ginger, jujube, bupleurum, licorice, cimicifuga

Uses: a tonic for physical strength, also named King of Combinations *(I-wang-tang)*; a tendency towards anemia; lack of vitality, fatigability, lassitude, anorexia, reduced gastrointestinal function; anemia, weak constitution; hemorrhoids, anal prolapse; gastric weakness; anorexia; hypotension; excessive sweating, night sweats; pulmonary tuberculosis, pleuritis; prevents emaciation in the summer, improves physical strength during convalescence

★ Ginseng and Atractylodes Formula *(Sheng-ling-pai- chu-san)* 参苓白朮散
Ho chi chu fang

Herbs: ginseng, hoelen, atractylodes, dioscorea, dolichos, lotus seed, platycodon, coix, cardamon, licorice

Effects: strengthens the digestive organs, nourishes the spleen and stomach, eliminates fluids and stagnancy, harmonizes *ch'i*

Uses: a weak gastrointestinal tract, emaciation, poor complexion, indigestion, vomiting or diarrhea, a tendency towards incessant diarrhea, anorexia, chronic gastritis, gastroptosis, chronic diarrhea, fermentative dyspepsia; a glandular constitution, defective development; lack of physical strength during convalescence, lassitude

★ **Ginseng and Ginger Combination** ***(Jen-sheng-tang)*** 人参湯

Shang han lun , Chin kuei yao lueh

Herbs: ginseng, licorice, atractylodes, ginger

Effects: improves digestion, absorption, metabolism

Uses: poor complexion, cold hands and feet, fatigability, polyuria, diarrhea; gastritis, gastroptosis, gastrectasia, gastric ulcer, gastricism, gastrointestinal weakness, gastric weakness; vomiting, hypersalivation, vomiting of pregnancy; intercostal neuralgia; hemorrhage due to weak conformation; hemoptysis

★ **Ginseng and Gypsum Combination** ***(Pai-hu-chia-jen-sheng-tang)*** 白虎加人参湯

Shang han lun, Chin kuei yao lueh

Herbs: anemarrhena, oryza, gypsum, licorice, ginseng

Uses: acute febrile diseases with thirst, dry throat; stroke; diabetes mellitus; eczema

★ Ginseng and Longan Combination ***(Kuei-pi-tang)***
歸脾湯

Chi sheng fang

Herbs: ginseng, astragalus, atractylodes, longan, zizyphus, *tang-kuei,* polygala, saussurea, licorice, hoelen, ginger, jujube

Uses: poor gastrointestinal tract, weak constitution, poor complexion, "flushing up"; hemorrhaging due to mental and physical overwork; anemia; amnesia; neurosis, neurasthenia, insomnia; anemia due to hemorrhaging; menoxenia, dysmenorrhea; menopausal neurosis, menopausal disorders; anorexia

★ Ginseng, Longan and Bupleurum Combination ***(Chia-wei-kuei-pi-tang)*** 加味歸脾湯

Cheng chih chuen sheng

Herbs: ginseng, atractylodes, hoelen, zizyphus, longan, astragalus, *tang-kuei*, polygala, licorice, saussurea, jujube, dried ginger, bupleurum, gardenia. Made by adding bupleurum and gardenia to Ginseng and Longan Combination *(Kuei-pi-tang).*

Uses: suitable for Ginseng and Longan conformation with fever; weakness of heart and spleen, pale complexion, weak constitution, weak pulse and abdomen, fatigability, neurosis, insomnia, mental instability, intestinal hemorrhaging, metrorrhagia, gastric ulcers, anemia and weakness due to hematuria, anorexia, neurasthenia, involuntary emissions

☆ **Ginseng and Mentha Formula *(Jen-sheng-pai-tu-san)*** 人參敗毒散

Ho chi chu fang

Herbs: ginseng, chianghuo, *tu-huo,* bupleurum, peucedanum, cnidium, *chih-ko*, pink hoelen, licorice, mentha, forsythia, lonicera

Effects: a dispersing agent used to remove summer fever, wet fever, pain in the limbs, stiffness in the neck

Uses: common cold, influenza, coughing, nasal congestion, urticaria, eczema

★ ☆ **Ginseng Nutritive Combination *(Jen-sheng-yang-yung-tang)*** 人參養榮湯

***Ho chi chu fang* (Formulas of Famous Physicians in the Sung Dynasty)**

Herbs: ginseng, *tang-kuei*, rehmannia, atractylodes, hoelen, cinnamon, peony, polygala, citrus, astragalus, licorice, schizandra

Effects: strengthens the body

Uses: a weak conformation; convalescence or following childbirth; tuberculosis; amnesia, baldness, general weakness, anemia, absence of facial luster, insomnia, cardiac hyperfunction, anorexia

★ ☆ Ginseng and *Tang-kuei* Ten Combination *(Shih-chuan-ta-pu-tang)* 十全大補湯
Ho chi chu fang

Herbs: ginseng, astragalus, atractylodes, *tang-kuei*, hoelen, rehmannia, cnidium, peony, cinnamon, licorice

Effects: nourishes *ch'i* and blood; strengthens weakness of yin, yang, surface, and interior

Uses: chronic diseases with general weakness, weakness during convalescence, fatigability, night sweats, cold hands and feet, anemia, anorexia, dry skin; after the onset of serious disease, surgery, childbirth; rheumatoid arthritis; "chill" abscess

☆ Ginseng and Zizyphus Formula *(Tien-wang-pu-hsin-tan)* 天王補心丹
Shih i teh hsiao fang

Herbs: rehmannia, ginseng, scrophularia, salvia root, hoelen, platycodon, polygala, zizyphus, biota, asparagus, ophiopogon, *tang-kuei*, schizandra, cinnabar, acorus

Effects: tranquilizes, nourishes blood and sperm

Uses: worry and anxiety, mental instability, involuntary emissions, amnesia, constipation, insomnia

☆ **Gleditsia Combination *(Tuo-li-hsiao-tu-yin)***
托裏消毒飲
Wan ping huei chun

Herbs: ginseng, cnidium, platycodon, atractylodes, peony, *tang-kuei*, hoelen, licorice, gleditsia, angelica, astragalus, lonicera

Effects: eliminates toxins, strengthens the body. For suppurative diseases in people of somewhat poor physical strength, it disperses toxin, improves pus expulsion, and speeds granulation; if vitality is very weak, Astragalus and Platycodon Formula *(Chien-chin-nei-tuo-san)* is used instead.

Uses: suppurative lymphadenitis, subepidermic abscess, carbuncles and furuncles, periproctitis

★ **Hoelen and Alisma Combination *(Fen-hsiao-tang)***
分消湯
Wan ping hui chun

Herbs: atractylodes, hoelen, white atractylodes, citrus, magnolia, cyperus, polyporus, alisma, *chih-shih*, areca, cardamon, saussurea, ginger, juncus

Effects: removes obstructions, smooths *ch'i*, eliminates food stagnancy and edema

Uses: for people of average physical strength in the initial stage of ascites with abdominal distention, edema, oliguria, nephritis, nephrosclerosis, peritonitis, or cirrhosis

★ Hoelen Five Herb Formula *(Wu-ling-san)* 五苓散
Shang han lun, Chin kuei yao lueh

Herbs: alisma, polyporus, hoelen, atractylodes, cinnamon

Effects: prevents hangover (called the drinker's friend)

Uses: faulty metabolism of fluid such as a dry mouth, oliguria, headache, abdominal pain, nausea and vomiting; children's common cold or autointoxication; nephritis; nephrosclerosis; nephropathy; thirst, abnormal urination, edema

★ Hoelen and Atractylodes Combination *(Ling-kuei-chu-kan-tang)* 苓桂朮甘湯
Shang han lun, Chin kuei yao lueh

Herbs: hoelen, cinnamon, atractylodes, licorice

Effects: stimulates the spirit and mind

Uses: dizziness, heavy headedness, orthostatic vertigo, tinnitus, cardiac asthma, palpitations, oliguria, abnormal heartbeat, cardiac asthma, mental abnormality, tinnitus, insomnia, pseudomyopia, eye fatigability, gasping, headache; most effective for chronic headache with vertigo

☆ **Hoelen and Schizandra Combination** ***(Ling-kan-chiang-wei-hsin-hsia-jen-tang)*** 苓甘薑味辛夏仁湯
Chin kuei yao lueh

Herbs: hoelen, pinellia, apricot seed, schizandra, licorice, ginger, asarum

Uses: weak and chill constitution with anemic asthmatic coughing; geriatric chronic bronchitis, asthma, and pulmonary emphysema; bronchial asthma; cardiac asthma; chronic nephritis

★ **Kaki Combination** ***(Shih-ti-tang)*** 柿蒂湯
Chi sheng fang

Herbs: clove, kaki, ginger

Uses: hiccoughs due to gastric chills (also cured by kaki alone)

★ **Baked Licorice Combination** ***(Chih-kan-tsao-tang)*** 炙甘草湯
Shang han lun, Chin kuei yao lueh

Herbs: baked licorice, ginger, cinnamon, jujube, linum, ginseng, rehmannia, ophiopogon, gelatin

Effects: stimulates the heart

Uses: irregular heartbeat, gasping, knotty and impeded pulse, weakness, fatigability; heart disease; cardiac hyperfunction; goiter

★ **Licorice and Jujube Combination** ***(Kan-mai-ta-tsao-tang)*** 甘麥大棗湯
Chin kuei yao lueh

Herbs: licorice, jujube, wheat

Effects: tranquilizes excessive nervous excitability. Alleviates impetuous spasms and hysteria in women but may be used regardless of sex or age.

Uses: depression without reason, crying over trivialities, insomnia, absent mindedness, frequent yawning, hysteria, chorea, night crying, epilepsy, spasms, nervous tic or twitching

★ **Licorice and Pinellia Combination** ***(Kan-tsao-hsieh-hsin-tang)*** 甘草瀉心湯
Shang han lun, Chin kuei yao lueh

Herbs: pinellia, scute, dried ginger, ginseng, jujube, licorice, coptis

Uses: for people of the Pinellia *(Pan-hsia-hsieh-hsin-tang)* conformation with mental instability, irrationality, gastroenteritis with a stagnant sensation below the sternum, severe diarrhea, stomatitis, bad breath, neurosis, or insomnia

☆ **Ludwigia Formula** ***(Teng-hua-pai-tu-san)***
燈花敗毒散
Sun-ten's formula

Herbs: ludwigia, pink hoelen, rhubarb, lithospermum, polygonum, polyporus, alisma, *Gleditsiae spina*, ginger

Effects: disinfects, reduces fever and inflammation, eases urination

Uses: the intitial stage of urticaria, itching

★ **Lithospermum Ointment** ***(Tzu-yun-kao)*** 紫雲膏
Hua kang ching chou

Herbs: sesame oil, *tang-kuei,* lithospermum, flava wax, lard

Effects: reduces fever and inflammation, arrests bleeding, kills pain, disinfects, strengthens the body

Uses: granulation, dry skin, chapping, ulceration, abnormal skin vegetation, suppuration, itching, burns, frigorism, injuries, knife wounds, hemorrhoids, inflammative boils, blemishes, perspiration sores, pain due to hemorrhoids, anal fissures

★ **Lotus Seed Combination** ***(Ching-hsin-lien-tzu-yin)***
清心蓮子飲
Ho chi chu fang

Herbs: lotus seed, ophiopogon, hoelen, ginseng, plantago, scute, astragalus, lycium bark, licorice

Uses: for people strong in the upper part of the body but weak in the lower; serious heart fever in the upper warmer, kidney weakness in the lower warmer; urinary disorders due to an insufficiency of harmony in the upper and lower warmers; frequent urination, turbid urine, involuntary emissions, a sensation of residual urine, leukorrhea, rough urination, painful urination, general lassitude, dry mouth and tongue; renal tuberculosis; chronic gonorrhea, chronic cystisis; urethritis; prostatomegaly; chronic pyelitis; sexual neurasthenia, impotence; diabetes mellitus; stomatitis

☆ **Lotus Stamen Formula** ***(Chin-sou-ku-ching-wan)***
金鎖固精丸
I fang chi chieh

Herbs: lotus seed, tribulus, euryale, lotus stamen, dragon bone, oyster shell

Effects: astringes, nourishes the body

Uses: involuntary emissions, enuresis, sexual neurasthenia

☆ **Lycium Formula *(Huan-shao-tan)*** 還少丹
Yang shih fang

Herbs: acorus, dioscorea, achyranthes, cornus, polygala, morinda, schizandra, cistanche, broussonetia, hoelen, lycium, rehmannia, fennel, eucommia, jujube

Effects: nourishes the meridians of the heart, kidney, spleen, and stomach

Uses: insufficiency of sperm and blood, spermatorrhea, anorexia, fever, night sweats, toothache, lower back pain, lassitude, weakness due to age, loss of sexual ability, reduced libido. Long term use makes one feel comfortable and look younger; for women, it is used as a cosmetic and to warm the uterus.

☆ **Magnolia Flower Formula *(Hsin-i-san)*** 辛夷散
Cheng chih chuen sheng

Herbs: magnolia flower, angelica, cimicifuga, *kao-pen*, siler, cnidium, asarum, akebia, licorice, *chianghuo*

Effects: removes obstructions

Uses: nasal congestion, chills in the head, incessant nasal drip, impaired sense of smell, common cold, headaches, nasal suppuration, chronic rhinitis

★ ☆ Magnolia and Ginger Formula ***(Ping-wei-san)***
平胃散
Ho chi chu fang

Herbs: atractylodes, magnolia, citrus, ginger, jujube, licorice

Uses: gastrointestinal disorders due to indigestion, borborygmus, diarrhea after meals, chronic and acute gastritis, gastric weakness, indigestion, anorexia

★ Magnolia Flower and Gypsum Combination ***(Hsin-i-ching-fei-tang)*** 辛夷清肺湯
Wai ko cheng tsung **(Principles of Surgery)**

Herbs: magnolia flower, eriobotrya, anemarrhena, lily, scute, ophiopogon, gypsum, cimicifuga, gardenia

Uses: pulmonary fever, nasal congestion, impaired sense of smell, feverish sensation in the nostrils, thirst, nasal suppuration, hypertrophic rhinitis, nasal polyps

★ *Ma-huang* Combination ***(Ma-huang-tang)*** 麻黄湯
Shang han lun

Herbs: *ma-huang*, apricot seed, cinnamon, licorice

Effects: stimulates perspiration and urination. After taking it, the patient feels more comfortable.

Uses: anhidrosis and general pain are the main symptoms; a weak cough, the initial stage of a common cold, fear of chills, fever, headache, common cold, asthma, rhinitis, runny nose

★ ***Ma-huang* and Apricot Seed Combination *(Ma-hsin-kan-shih-tang)*** 麻杏甘石湯
Shang han lun

Herbs: *ma-huang*, apricot seed, licorice, gypsum

Uses: attacks of bronchial asthma, especially in children; severe cough, heavy sweating, and dry mouth during asthmatic attacks; bronchitis; children's asthma; whooping cough

☆ ***Ma-huang* and Asarum Combination *(Ma-huang-hsi-hsin-fu-tzu-tang)*** 麻黄細辛附子湯
Shang han lun

Herbs: *ma-huang*, asarum, aconite

Uses: external sensations of a weak constitution—fever, fear of chills, chills in the hands and feet, pain in the loin and back; common cold in weak or elderly people; bronchitis, bronchial asthma

☆ ***Ma-huang* and Cimicifuga Combination *(Shih-shen-tang)* 十神湯**

Ho chi chu fang

Herbs: cnidium, licorice, *ma-huang*, perilla, angelica, cimicifuga, citrus, cyperus, peony, jujube, pueraria, ginger

Uses: common cold, headaches, fever, fear of chills, absence of sweating, coughing

★ ***Ma-huang* and Coix Combination *(Ma-hsin-i-kan-tang)* 麻杏薏甘湯**

Chin kuei yao lueh

Herbs: *ma-huang*, apricot seed, coix, licorice

Uses: rheumatalgia, acute or chronic; for people who have pain when the weather turns cold—arthritis, neuralgia, muscle pain

☆ ***Ma-huang* and Ginkgo Combination *(Ting-chuan-tang)* 定喘湯**

I fang chi chieh

Herbs: *ma-huang*, pinellia, apricot seed, scute, licorice, gingko, tussilago, morus, perilla fruit

Effects: dispels sputum, arrests asthma

Uses: asthma with coughing, mucous sound in the throat, instability, anorexia, bronchitis, bronchial asthma, asthma

★ *Ma-huang* and Ginseng Combination *(Hsu-ming-tang)* 續命湯
Chin kuei yao lueh

Herbs: apricot seed, *ma-huang*, cinnamon, ginseng, *tang-kuei*, cnidium, ginger, licorice, gypsum

Uses: hemiplegia, hoarseness due to apoplexy, headaches, stridor, thirst, dyskinesia, hoarseness, hypertension, cerebromalacia, hemiplegia due to an apopletic seizure

★ *Ma-huang* and Magnolia Combination *(Shen-mi-tang)* 神秘湯
Wai tai mi yao

Herbs: *ma-huang*, apricot seed, magnolia, citrus, licorice, bupleurum, perilla

Uses: labored breathing with little sputum, bronchial asthma complicated by anxiety, children's asthma

☆ ***Ma-huang* and Morus Formula *(Hua-kai-san)*** 華蓋散
Ho chi chu fang

Herbs: *ma-huang,* morus, perilla fruit, apricot seed, hoelen, citrus, licorice. An altered form of *Ma-huang* Combination *(Ma-huang-tang).*

Uses: asthmatic cough, weak gastrointestinal tract, children's asthmatic cough, common cold, bronchitis, bronchial asthma, whooping cough

★ **Major Bupleurum Combination *(Ta-chai-hu-tang)***
大柴胡湯
Shang han lun*, *Chin kuei yao lueh

Herbs: bupleurum, pinellia, ginger, scute, peony, jujube, *chih-shih*, rhubarb

Uses: for people past middle age with a strong physique and average strength, a tendency toward constipation, insomnia, fatigability, lassitude, and loss of energy; cholelithiasis; cholecystitis; hepatitis; gastritis; hypertension; obesity; habitual constipation; shoulder stiffness; headache due to hypertension

★ Major Zanthoxylum Combination ***(Ta-chien-chung-tang)*** 大建中湯

Chin kuei yao lueh

Herbs: zanthoxylum, ginseng, ginger, maltose

Uses: paroxysmal intestinal hyperperistalsis with a weak and chill condition and severe abdominal pain; chilling pain in the abdomen; abdominal distention; intestinal colic; abdominal pain due to ascarides; localized peritonitis

★ Minor Blue Dragon Combination ***(Hsiao-ching-lung-tang)*** 小青龍湯

Shang han lun, Chin kuei yao lueh

Herbs: *ma-huang*, peony, ginger, licorice, cinnamon, asarum, pinellia, schizandra

Effects: eliminates congestion and cough, eases urination

Uses: cough and asthma due to common cold and bronchitis, common cold, allergic rhinitis, bronchitis, bronchial asthma, whooping cough, runny nose, cough with watery sputum, tearing

★ **Minor Bupleurum Combination** ***(Hsiao-chai-hu-tang)*** 小柴胡湯
Shang han lun, Chin kuei yao lueh

Herbs: bupleurum, pinellia, ginger, scute, jujube, ginseng, licorice

Uses: for people at the onset of illness with anorexia and lassitude and white tongue fur with mild fever or vomiting and nausea; common cold or feverish diseases; severe common cold; bronchitis; gastric weakness, gastroenteritis; liver disease; lymphadenitis; pulmonary tuberculosis; pleuritis

★ **Minor Cinnamon and Peony Combination** ***(Hsiao-chien-chung-tang)*** 小建中湯

Herbs: cinnamon, ginger, jujube, peony, licorice, maltose

Uses: a weak constitution; poor complexion, abdominal pain, palpitations, fever in the hands and feet, chills, frequent urination and polyuria; as a tonic for the development of body and brain in debilitated children with enuresis and night crying; abdominal pain; hernia; constipation

★ **Minor Pinellia and Hoelen Combination** ***(Hsiao-pan-hsia-chia-fu-ling-tang)*** 小半夏加茯苓湯
Chin kuei yao lueh

Herbs: pinellia, ginger, hoelen

Uses: pregnant vomiting, incessant vomiting due to illness, nausea

Morus and Chrysanthemum Combination ***(Sang-chu-yin)*** 桑菊飲
Wen ping tiao pien

Herbs: morus leaves, apricot seed, forsythia, mentha, chrysanthemum, platycodon, licorice, phragmites

Uses: the initial stage of an acute febrile disease, fever, cough, mild thirst, common cold, headache, vertigo

☆ **Musk and Catechu Formula** ***(Chi-li-san)*** 七厘散
An experimental formula

Herbs: calamus gum, mastic, myrrh, carthamus, catechu, cinnabar, musk, borneol

Uses: contusions, stagnant occluded blood, general pain

★ Ophiopogon Combination ***(Mai-men-tung-tang)***
麥門冬湯
Chin kuei yao lueh

Herbs: ophiopogon, oryza, pinellia, jujube, ginseng, licorice

Uses: spasmodic coughing due to flushing up of *ch'i*, a dry throat, cough with scanty sputum, hoarseness, bronchitis, asthma, whooping cough, loss of voice

★ Ophiopogon and Asarum Combination ***(Ching-shang-chuan-tung-tang)*** 清上蠲痛湯
Shou shih pao yuan

Herbs: tang-kuei, **cnidium, chianghuo,** ***tu-huo*****, siler, atractylodes, ophiopogon, scute, chrysanthemum, vitex, asarum, licorice, ginger, angelica**

Uses: chronic headaches, headaches, facial pain, trifacial neuralgia, pain due to cancer of the upper jaw

☆ Peony and Licorice Combination ***(Shao-yao-kan-tsao-tang)*** 芍藥甘草湯
Shang han lun

Herbs: peony, licorice

Effects: eliminates pain in the limbs, colic pain due to kidney stones, or biliary calculi

Uses: acute muscular spasms and pain, spasms and pain in the hands and feet due to excessive exercise, severe pain due to dysmenorrhea, pain from kidney stones and biliary calculi

★ **Persica and Rhubarb Combination *(Tao-ho-cheng-chi-tang)*** 桃核承氣湯
Shang han lun, Chin kuei yao lueh

Herbs: persica, cinnamon, mirabilitum, rhubarb, licorice

Effects: dispels occluded blood

Uses: red and dark facial complexion with headaches, dizziness, chills in the lower abdomen, lumbago, constipation and menoxenia; also advisable for urinary retention due to contusion, habitual constipation, freckles, eczema, disorders due to menoxenia, menopausal disorders, and neuralgia

★ **Phellodendron Combination *(Tzu-yin-chiang-huo-iang)*** 滋陰降火湯
Wan ping huei chun

Herbs: *tang-kuei*, peony, rehmannia, asparagus, ophiopogon, citrus, atractylodes, anemarrhena, phellodendron, licorice

Uses: lack of body fluids, dry throat, palpitations, gasping, thirst, insomnia, vegetative pulmonary tuberculosis, dry pleuritis, bronchitis, pyelitis, diabetes mellitus

Pinellia and Gardenia Combination *(Li-ke-tang)*
利膈湯

Japanese formula

Herbs: pinellia, aconite, gardenia

Uses: stenosis in the throat and esophagus, a sensation of obstruction, difficulty swallowing, vomiting, sticky sputum, thirst, esophageal spasms, esophageal carcinoma or tumor, obstruction of the throat, gastric cancer

★ Pinellia Combination *(Pan-hsia-hsieh-hsin-tang)*
半夏瀉心湯

Shang han lun, Chin kuei yao lueh

Herbs: pinellia, scute, coptis, ginseng, jujube, ginger, licorice. As famous as Cardamon and Fennel Formula *(An-chung-san)* for gastrointestinal disorders.

Uses: stagnancy below the sternum, borborygmus, diarrhea with gastritis, gastroptosis, and chronic dysentery; alternating diarrhea and constipation, or nausea, vomiting, and anorexia; gastrectasia; gastric ulcer; fermentative diarrhea

★ **Pinellia and Gastrodia Combination *(Pan-hsia-pai-chu-tien-ma-tang)*** 半夏白朮天麻湯

Pi wei lun

Herbs: pinellia, atractylodes, citrus, hoelen, malt, gastrodia, ginger, *shen-chu*, astragalus, ginseng, alisma, phellodendron, dried ginger

Effects: nourishes the spleen and stomach, eases urination, removes stagnant water from the stomach

Uses: weak gastrointestinal tract with paroxysmal headaches and vertigo, chills in the legs and feet, gastric atonia, gastroptosis, gastritis, neurosis, hypertension, suppuration

★ **Pinellia and Ginger Combination *(Sheng-chiang-hsieh-hsin-tang)*** 生薑瀉心湯

Shang han lun, Chin kuei yao lueh

Herbs: pinellia, scute, dried ginger, ginseng, licorice, jujube, coptis, ginger

Uses: for people of a Pinellia *(Pan-hsia-hsieh-hsin-tang)* conformation with a stagnant sensation below the sternum, belching, and fetid odor caused by fermentation of stagnant food in the stomach (ginger improves digestion); gastritis; gastrosia; fermentative diarrhea; anorexia; vomiting; bad breath

☆ Pinellia and Ginseng Six Combination *(Pan-hsieh-liu-chun-tzu-tang)* 半瀉六君子湯

Herbs: pinellia, ginseng, scute, hoelen, oyster shell, ginger, atractylodes, coptis, licorice, citrus

Uses: stagnant heaviness in the stomach with nausea, stomachache when hungry, and general malnutrition; gastroenteritis; gastric ulcers; gastroptosis; stomachache; gastric spasms; abdominal pain; duodenal ulcers; an emaciated constitution

★ Pinellia and Magnolia Combination *(Pan-hsia-hou-pu-tang)* 半夏厚朴湯

Chin kuei yao lueh

Herbs: pinellia, hoelen, ginger, magnolia, perilla

Uses: neurosis, daydreaming, mental instability due to nervousness and anxiety; blocked *ch'i*, a sensation of a foreign body in the throat and esophagus; palpitations, vertigo, nausea; neurasthenia, mental abnormality; bronchitis, bronchial asthma; neurotic esophageal stenosis; neurotic gastritis; pregnant vomiting; coughing and hoarseness

★ Platycodon and Coix Combination ***(Chieh-keng-tang)*** 桔梗湯

Wai tai mi yao

Herbs: platycodon, rehmannia, *tang-kuei*, licorice, thlaspi, morus, coix, saussurea

Uses: chronic pulmonary carbuncles, loss of vitality and blood, swelling and pain in the throat, leukorrhea, tonsillitis, peritonsillitis

★ Platycodon and Fritillary Combination ***(Ching-fei-tang)*** 清肺湯

Wan ping huei chun

Herbs: scute, platycodon, hoelen, citrus, *tang-kuei*, fritillary, morus, ophiopogon, asparagus, gardenia, apricot seed, schizandra, licorice, jujube, bamboo, ginger

Effects: nourishes the lungs, eliminates fever and sputum

Uses: cough, fever in the lungs, copious sputum, persistent cough; bronchitis, bronchiectasis

★ Polyporus Combination *(Chu-ling-tang)* 豬苓湯
Shang han lun, Chin kuei yao lueh

Herbs: polyporus, hoelen, alisma, gelatin, talcum

Uses: irregular urination, decreased urinary volume, painful urination, hematuria, a sensation of residual urine; nephritis, cystitis, urethritis, gallstones

★ Pueraria Combination *(Ko-ken-tang)* 葛根湯
Shang han lun

Herbs: pueraria, *ma-huang*, ginger, cinnamon, peony, licorice, jujube

Uses: excessive sweating, fear of chills, stiffness and spasms in the neck and back; common cold, runny nose; headaches; shoulder stiffness; muscle pain; pain in the hands and shoulders; inflammation; nasal suppuration; neuralgia; eczema; acute colitis; pimples, boils; tonsillitis, sore throat; mastitis, otitis media, loss of hearing; pyorrhea alveolaris; hordeolum, keratitis, iritis; fever; paralysis, spasms, lower back pain

★ Pueraria and Magnolia Flower Combination *(Ko-ken-tang-chia-chuan-chiung-hsin-i)* 葛根湯加川芎辛夷

Japanese formula

Herbs: pueraria, *ma-huang*, cinnamon, peony, jujube, ginger, licorice, cnidium, magnolia flower

Uses: nasal suppuration, chronic rhinitis, nasal congestion, common cold

★ **Pueraria, Coptis, and Scute Combination** ***(Ko-ken-huang-lien-huang-chin-tang)*** 葛根黃連黃芩湯
Shang han lun

Herbs: pueraria, coptis, scute, licorice

Uses: diarrhea, fever, shoulder stiffness; vomiting due to overdrinking; acute gastritis; colitis; infectious diarrhea; hypertension; common cold with gastrointestinal symptoms; stomatitis, inflammation of the tongue; insomnia

☆ **Pueraria Nasal Combination** ***(Ching- pi-tang)*** 清鼻湯
Chang tsang yen fang

Herbs: pueraria, cnidium, *ma-huang*, rhubarb, cinnamon bark, licorice, peony, coix, ginger, platycodon, gypsum, magnolia flower, jujube

Uses: nasal suppuration with heavy headedness, mental instability, and amnesia; inability to concentrate; chronic rhinitis, nasal congestion

★ ☆ Rehmannia Eight Formula *(Pa-wei-ti-huang-wan)* 八味地黄丸
Chin kuei yao lueh

Herbs: rehmannia, cornus, dioscorea, alisma, hoelen, moutan, cinnamon, aconite

Uses: fatigability, cold arms and legs, oliguria or polyuria, thirst, pain in the legs and feet, lower back pain, paralysis, presbyopia, itching, dysuria, frequent urination, edema, loss of energy—especially impotence, diabetes mellitus, geriatric pruritus, hypertension, neurasthenia, itching, cataracts, paralysis in the legs and feet, cystitis

★ ☆ Rehmannia Six Formula *(Liu-wei-ti-huang-wan)* 六味地黄丸
Chien i fang

Herbs: rehmannia, hoelen, moutan, alisma, dioscorea, cornus

Uses: low back pain and weak feet due to renal weakness, vertigo, emissions, urinary stuttering; diabetes mellitus; geriatric diseases; impotence, emissions; nephritis; dysuria, frequent urination; edema; cataracts, glaucoma. When used for fatigability, oliguria or polyuria, and thirst, the patient's condition is not as serious as for Rehmannia Eight Formula *(Pa-wei-ti-huang-wan)*.

★ **Rhubarb and Moutan Combination *(Ta-huang-mu-tan-pi-tang)*** 大黃牡丹皮湯
Chin kuei yao lueh

Herbs: rhubarb, moutan, persica, mirabilitum, benincasa

Effects: an exsanguinative for people of average physical strength

Uses: inflammation in the lower abdomen, a tendency towards constipation, appendicitis, uterine myoma, dysmenorrhea, irregular menstruation, ovaritis, pyelitis, hemorrhoids

★ **Schizonepeta and Forsythia Combination *(Ching-chieh-lien-chiao-tang)*** 荊芥連翹湯
Wan ping huei chun

Herbs: *tang-kuei*, peony, cnidium, scute, gardenia, forsythia, siler, schizonepeta, *chih-ko*, platycodon, angelica, bupleurum, licorice

Effects: improves the poison relieving constitution and an adenosis constitution

Uses: ear, nose, suppurative diseases; especially for people with mildly darkened skin and sweaty palms and soles; otitis media, nasal suppuration, rhinitis, chronic tonsillitis, acne

★ Schizonepeta and Siler Formula *(Ching-fang-pai-tu-san)* 荊防敗毒散

Wan ping huei chun

Herbs: schizonepeta, siler, chianghuo, *tu-huo,* bupleurum, peucedanum, mentha, forsythia, platycodon, *chih-ko*, cnidium, lonicera, licorice, ginger

Uses: suppurative diseases—the initial stage of fear of chills, fever, reddening, swelling, and pain; carbuncles and furunculosis; urticaria; eczema; scabies; head boils; nasal suppuration; dermatosis

Scute Combination *(Tzu-shen-tung-erh-tang)* 滋腎通耳湯

Wan ping huei chun

Herbs: *tang-kuei*, cnidium, peony, anemarrhena, rehmannia, phellodendron, scute, bupleurum, angelica, cyperus

Uses: tinnitus, dysacousia due to kidney weakness, hearing loss from otitis media, geriatric hearing loss, hearing loss due to medication

★ Scute and Coptis Combination *(Huang-lien-chieh-tu-tang)* 黄連解毒湯
Chou hou fang

Herbs: coptis, scute, phellodendron, gardenia

Effects: unblocks occluded blood, tranquilizes, and arrests bleeding in hemoptysis, nosebleeds, and hemorrhoidal hemorrhaging

Uses: people of average physical strength with a tendency towards flushing up, red complexion, mental instability, metrorrhagia, hypertension, stomatitis, and chest pain

★ Siler Combination *(Ching-shang-fang-feng-tang)* 清上防風湯
Wan ping huei chun

Herbs: siler, forsythia, platycodon, angelica, scute, cnidium, schizonepeta, gardenia, coptis, mentha, *chih-ko*, licorice

Effects: dissipates firm fever

Uses: fever in the upper warmer with head boils; acne; eczema on the head; acne rosacea; and as a cosmetic

★ ☆ Siler and Platycodon Formula *(Fang-feng-tung-sheng-san)* 防風通聖散

Hsuan ming lun

Herbs: *tang-kuei*, peony, cnidium, gardenia, forsythia, mentha, ginger, schizonepeta, siler, *ma-huang*, rhubarb, mirabilitum, platycodon, scute, gypsum, licorice, talcum, atractylodes

Effects: improves the constitution, reduces weight

Uses: for stout people with subepidermal lipomatosis in the abdomen, periodic constipation or habitual constipation, cardiac weakness, arteriosclerosis, apoplexy, nephritis, and complications of hypertension such as palpitations, shoulder stiffness and flushing up; edema

☆★ Six Major Herb Combination *(Liu-chun-tzu-tang)* 六君子湯

Wan ping huei chun

Herbs: ginseng, atractylodes, hoelen, pinellia, citrus, ginger, jujube, licorice

Uses: gastrointestinal weakness, food stagnancy with anorexia, nausea, stagnancy and fullness below the sternum, cold hands and feet due to anemia, fatigability, gastrectasia, gastroptosis, chronic gastroenteritis, gastritis, gastric weakness, dyspepsia, stomachache, vomiting, an emaciated constitution

★ **Stephania and Astragalus Combination *(Fang-chi-huang-chi-tang)*** 防己黃耆湯
Chin kuei yao lueh

Herbs: stephania, astragalus, atractylodes, ginger, jujube, licorice

Uses: mostly for obese women with white skin, soft muscles, fatigability, excessives sweating, rheumatic arthritis, muscle pain, uratic (gouty) arthritis, rheumatism, arthritis, and edema

☆ **Stephania and Ginseng Combination *(Mu-fang-chi-tang)*** 木防己湯
Chin kuei yao lueh

Herbs: stephania, gypsum, cinnamon, ginseng

Uses: stagnancy and hardening beneath the heart, insufficiency of cardiac function with edema and oliguria, valvular disease, cardiac asthma, nephritis

☆ **Sweet Combination *(Kan-lu-yin)*** 甘露飲
Ho chi chu fang

Herbs: eriobotrya, asparagus, *chih-shih*, capillaris, ophiopogon, dendrobium, licorice, scute, rehmannia

Uses: wet fever in the digestive organs; swelling and erosion of the mouth, tongue, gingiva, and throat with pus and blood; gingivitis; pyorrhea alveolaris; stomatitis; scurvy

★ ***Tang-kuei* Combination *(Tang-kuei-tang)* 當歸湯**
Chien chin fang

Herbs: *tang-kuei*, pinellia, peony, magnolia, cinnamon, ginseng, ginger, astragalus, zanthoxylum, licorice

Uses: poor complexion, chills in the back, acute chest pain, weakness, abdominal distention and pain, thoracic neuralgia, angina pectoris, gastric and duodenal ulcers

***Tang-kuei* and Anemarrhena Combination *(Tang-kuei-nien-tung-tang)* 當歸拈痛湯**
Lan shih mi tsang

Herbs: *tang-kuei,* anemarrhena, chianghuo, capillaris, scute, angelica, polyporus, alisma, atractylodes, siler, pueraria, ginseng, sophora, cimicifuga, licorice

Uses: reddening and swelling pain of the joints due to wet fever; general pain; painful swelling in the ankle; boils; reddening and swelling with pus and water; reddening and painful swelling in the joints; arthritis; dermatosis in the legs and feet; beriberi

★ ***Tang-kuei* and Arctium Formula *(Hsiao-feng-san)***
消風散

Wai ko cheng tsung

Herbs: *tang-kuei*, rehmannia, gypsum, siler, atractylodes, arctium, akebia, anemarrhena, sesame, sophora, schizonepeta, cicada, licorice

Uses: internal fever, copious secretion, skin disease with severe itching. Most effective for eczema which worsens in summer with discharge and crusting; chronic eczema (with copious discharge); and urticaria

★ ***Tang-kuei* , Astragalus, and Peony Combination *(Kuei-chi- chien-chung-tang)*** 歸耆建中湯

Japanese formula

Herbs: *tang-kuei*, cinnamon, ginger, jujube, peony, licorice, astragalus, maltose. Astragalus Combination *(Huang-chi-chien-chung-tang)* is made by adding astragalus to Minor Cinnamon and Peony Combination *(Hsiao-chien-chung-tang)*; if *tang-kuei* is added to Astragalus Combination, *Tang-kuei*, Astragalus, and Peony Combination results.

Uses: blood weakness external and internal; weak constitution, weakness during convalescence; night sweats, anal fistula, hemorrhoids, chronic otitis media, chronic ulcers, suppurative abcess

☆ ***Tang-kuei* and Eight Herb Formula *(Pa-wei-tai-hsia-fang)*** 八味帶下方
Ming chia fang hsuan

Herbs: smilax, *tang-kuei*, cnidium, akebia, hoelen, citrus, lonicera, rhubarb

Uses: leukorrhea without severe inflammation or congestion, chronic leukorrhea, suppurative leukorrhea with a fetid odor, gonococcal leukorrhea

★ ***Tang-kuei* and Evodia Combination *(Wen-ching-tang)*** 溫經湯
Chin kuei yao lueh

Herbs: evodia, *tang-kuei*, cnidium, peony, ginseng, cinnamon, gelatin, moutan, ginger, licorice, pinellia, ophiopogon

Uses: women's diseases with weak *ch'i* and blood, chills, annoying fever in the palms, and dry mouth and lips; menoxenia; infertility; menopausal disorders; abnormal leukorrhea; eczema; keratosis of the palm; insomnia; neurosis; chills in the feet and loin; frigorism

★ *Tang-kuei*, Evodia and Ginger Combination *(Tang-kuei-szu-ni-chia-wu-chu-yu-sheng-chiang-tang)*
當歸四逆加吳茱萸生薑湯
Shang han lun, Chin kuei yao lueh

Herbs: *tang-kuei*, cinnamon, peony, akebia, ginger, asarum, licorice, evodia, jujube

Effects: prevents frigorism and exacerbation of pain during cold weather, warms the blood, improves circulation in the extremeties

Uses: chills, cold hands and feet, cold legs and feet with pain, frigorism, headaches, pain in the legs and feet or lower abdomen, lower back pain, neuralgia, dysmenorrhea, abdominal pain due to uterine or ovarian disease

★ *Tang-kuei* Four Combination *(Szu-wu-tang)* 四物湯
Ho chi chu fang

Herbs: *tang-kuei*, cnidium, peony, rehmannia

Effects: nourishes the blood, aids manufacture of blood, tranquilizes, strengthens the heart

Uses: for people with dry skin and a poor complexion without gastrointestinal disorders; mostly for women's diseases but can be used by men; onset of disease; before or after childbirth; fatigability after childbirth or abortion; menoxenia; infertility;

frigorism; chills; menopausal neuralgia, menopausal disorders

★ ***Tang-kuei* and Gambir Combination *(Chi-wu-chiang-hsia-tang)*** 七物降下湯

A Japanese formula from Keisetsu Otsuka

Herbs: *tang-kuei*, peony, rehmannia, cnidium, phellodendron, astragalus, gambir

Uses: a weak conformation with hypertension; a tendency towards emaciation with hypertension, "flushing up," shoulder stiffness, tinnitus, a heavy head; kidney disorders, hypertension due to kidney disorders, chronic nephritis; arteriosclerosis

★ ***Tang-kuei* and Gardenia Combination *(Wen-ching-yin)*** 溫清飲

Wan ping huei chun

Herbs: *tang-kuei*, rehmannia, peony, cnidium, coptis, scute, phellodendron, gardenia. A combined form of *Tang-kuei* Four Combination *(Szu-ni-tang)* and Scute and Coptis Combination *(Huang-lien-chieh-tu-tang)*.

Uses: for people of anemic constitution with skin disease, eczema, poor complexion, "flushing up," hemorrhaging, metrorrhagia, anemia, dermatosis, melasma, menopausal neurosis, neurosis

★ *Tang-kuei* and Gelatin Combination *(Chiung-kuei-chiao-ai-tang)* 芎歸膠艾湯
Chin kuei yao lueh

Herbs: cnidium, licorice, artemisia, gelatin, *tang-kuei,* peony, rehmannia

Effects: stops hemorrhaging, strengthens the body

Uses: metrorrhagia, hemorrhoidal hemorrhaging, signs of abortion, hematuria, postpartum hemorrhaging, anemia, hemorrhaging in the lower abdomen—any kind of hemorrhage; anemia in women from persistent bleeding

☆ *Tang-kuei* and Ginger Combination *(Sheng-hua-tang)* 生化湯
Fu ching chu nu ko

Herbs: *tang-kuei*, cnidium, persica, ginger, licorice

Effects: administered two or three days after childbirth; removes obstructions, nourishes the body, eliminates occluded blood

Uses: as a tonic for the body and blood; postpartum abdominal pain, the absence of lochia

★ *Tang-kuei* and Magnolia Formula *(Wu-chi-san)*
五積散
Ho chi chu fang

Herbs: hoelen, white atractylodes, citrus, pinellia, atractylodes, *tang-kuei*, peony, cnidium, magnolia, angelica, *chih-ko*, platycodon, ginger, cyperus, cinnamon, *ma-huang*, jujube, licorice

Uses: stagnant *ch'i*, blood, sputum and food with chills; for people with a weak liver and spleen and disease due to chills and wetness; anemia; fever in the upper body and chills in the lower body; lumbago due to chills; spasms in the lumbar region, pain in the lower abdomen; gastroenteritis; neuralgia; arthritis; menorrhalgia; chills; menopausal disorders; common cold; gastric ulcers, duodenal ulcers; gastric spasms, hernia; sciatica

☆ *Tang-kuei* and Parsley Combination *(Pao-chan-wu-yu-fang)* 保產無憂方
Pu i fang

Herbs: magnolia, artemisia, cnidium, *tang-kuei*, schizonepeta, fritillaria, cuscuta, chianghuo, licorice, *chih-ko*, peony, ginger, astragalus

Effects: also named "thirteen odors"; a tonic before childbirth—nourishes the blood, tranquilizes the fetus. It may be administered after the middle stage of pregnancy to tranquilize the fetus and hasten birth.

Uses: vomiting sputum and water during pregnancy, fear of the smell of food, sore loins and abdominal pain, fetal movement and instability, incessant hemorrhaging

★ *Tang-kuei* and Peony Formula *(Tang-kuei-shao-yao-san)* 當歸芍藥散
Chin kuei yao lueh

Herbs: *tang-kuei*, cnidium, peony, hoelen, atractylodes, alisma

Effects: improves blood circulation, tranquilizes the fetus

Uses: a tonic for women of chillphobic constitution with anemia and for people of poor physical strength with chills, a tendency towards anemia, fatigability, pain in the lower abdomen, heavy headedness, vertigo, shoulder stiffness, tinnitus, and palpitations; a tonic for women with menoxenia and disorders caused by pregnancy, childbirth, or abortion—anemia, fatigability, vertigo, edema; lower back pain; chills in the feet and loin; habitual spontaneous abortion; infertility; chills; frigorism; keratosis of the palm

☆ ***Tu-huo*** **and Vaeicum Combination** ***(Tu-huo-chi-sheng-tang)*** 獨活寄生湯
Chien chin fang

Herbs: *tu-huo*, loranthus, *chin-chiu*, siler, asarum, *tang-kuei*, peony, cnidium, rehmannia, eucommia, achyranthes, ginseng, hoelen, licorice, cinnamon bark

Effects: improves blood circulation, stops pain, reduces paralysis

Uses: osseous rheumatic neuralgia due to a weak conformation; pain in the loin and back during pregnancy; lower back pain; pain or numbness in the knees and feet; neuralgia; rheumatism. Not suitable for acute rheumatism.

★ **Vitality Combination** ***(Chen-wu-tang)*** 眞武湯
Shang han lun, Chin kuei yao lueh

Herbs: hoelen, peony, ginger, atractylodes, aconite

Uses: disease caused by faulty metabolism, i.e., excessive sweating, vertigo, palpitations, chills in the limbs, diarrhea; chronic diarrhea; gastrointestinal weakness; febrile diseases; peritonitis; appendicitis

☆ **WTTC** ***(Lo-shih-shu)*** 樂適舒
Chang tsang yen fang

Herbs: coix, terminalia, trapa, wisteria

Effects: 20% effective for gastric cancer and rectal cancer; inhibits growth of cancer cells, prevents metastasis after surgery; reduces fever, inflammation, pain, and spasms; eases urination

Uses: edema, arthralgia, gastric cancer

☆ **Xanthium Formula** ***(Tsang-erh-san)*** 蒼耳散
Cheng chih chuen sheng

Herbs: xanthium, magnolia flower, angelica, mentha

Uses: nasal suppuration, chronic rhinitis

★ **Zizyphus Combination** ***(Suan-tsao-jen-tang)***
酸棗仁湯
Chin kuei yao lueh

Herbs: zizyphus, hoelen, anemarrhena, cnidium, licorice

Uses: insomnia due to mental and physical exhaustion or weakness, general insomnia, night sweats, amnesia

V. APPENDIX OF HERBS AND THEIR USES

Chinese Name (Alpha Name)	Common Name	Part Used	Scientific Name (Family Name)	Medical Uses
五加皮 (Wu-chia-pi)	Acanthopanax	Root epidermis	*Acanthopanax gracilistylus* W. W. Smith (Araliaceae)	Antirheumatic, restoring vigor and sexual potency
牛膝 (Niu-hsi)	Achyranthes	Root	*Achyranthes bidentata* Blume (Amaranthaceae)	Diuretic, emmenagogue, mucilaginous, demulcent

Chinese Name (Alpha Name)	Common Name	Part Used	Scientific Name (Family Name)	Medical Uses
附子 (Fu-tzu)	Aconite	Root	*Aconitum carmichaeli* Debx. (Ranunculaceae)	Stimulant, cardio-tonic, analgesic
石菖蒲 (Shih-chang-pu)	Acorus	Rhizome	*Acorus gramineus* Soland. (Araceae)	Stomachic in dyspepsia, hyperacidity
木通 (Mu-tang)	Akebia	Stem	*Akebia quinata Decne;* (Ranunculaceae) *Clematis armandi* Franch. (Lardizabalaceae)	Diuretic, antiphlogistic
澤瀉 (Tse-hsieh)	Alisma	Tuber	*Alisma plantago L.* (Alismataceae)	Diuretic, diaphoretic

Chinese Name (Alpha Name)	Common Name	Part Used	Scientific Name (Family Name)	Medical Uses
九節菖蒲 (Chiu-chieh-chang-pu)	Altaica	Rhizome	*Anemone altaica* Fisch. (Ranunculaceae)	Stimulant, expectorant, detoxifier
明礬 (Ming-fan)	Alum	Mineral	$KA1_3\ (SO_4)_2 \cdot 12H_2O$	Astringent, hemostatic, anthelminitic, detoxifier
知母 (Chih-mu)	Anemarrhena	Rhizome	*Anemarrhena asphodeloides* Bunge. (Liliaceae)	Antipyretic, expectorant
白頭翁 (Pai-tou-weng)	Anemone	Root	*Anemone cernua* Thunb., *A. pulsatilla* (Ranunculaceae)	Antidiarrheic

Chinese Name (Alpha Name)	Common Name	Part Used	Scientific Name (Family Name)	Medical Uses
白芷 (Pai-chih) (Tang-kuei)	Angelica	Root	*Angelica dahurica* var. *pai-chi; Angelica dahurica* Benth. et Hook. (Umbelliferae)	Aromatic, stimulant, analgesic
穿山甲 (Chuan-shan-chia)	Anteater Scales	Scales	*Manis pentadactyla* L. (Manidae)	Stimulate circulation, dispel pus
羚羊角 (Ling-yang-chueh)	Antelope Horn	Horn	*Saiga tatarica* L. *Nemorhaedus cripus* (Bovidae)	Antispasmodic, antipyretic, tonic
杏仁 (Hsing-jen)	Apricot Seed (Almond)	Seed	*Prunus armeniaca* L. (Rosaceae)	Antitussive, sedative in bronchitis, asthma

Chinese Name (Alpha Name)	Common Name	Part Used	Scientific Name (Family Name)	Medical Uses
沈香 (Shen-hsiang)	Aquilaria	Wood	*Aquilaria agallocha* Roxb. (Thymelaeaceae)	Stomachic in gastralgia, colic, nervous emesis
牛蒡子 (Niu-pang-tzu)	Arctium	Fruit	*Arctium lappa* L. (Compositae)	Diuretic, antipyretic, expectorant, antiphlogistic
大腹皮 (Ta-fu-pi)	Areca	Fruit rind	*Areca catechu* L. (Palmae)	Diuretic
檳榔 (Pin-lang)	Areca Seed	Seed	*Areca catechu* L. (Palmae)	Astringent taeniafuga

Chinese Name (Alpha Name)	Common Name	Part Used	Scientific Name (Family Name)	Medical Uses
天南星 (Tien-nan-hsing)	Arisaema	Tuber	*Arisaema amurense* Maximowicz (Araceae)	Analgesic, antispasmodic, taeniafuge
馬兜鈴 (Ma-tou-ling)	Aristolochia (Birthwort)	Fruit	*Aristolochia contorta* Bunge; *A. debilis* Sieb. et Zucc. (Aristolochiaceae)	Expectorant, antitussive
艾葉 (Ai-yeh)	Artemisia (Mugwort)	Leaves	*Artemisia vulgaris* L. (Compositae)	Hemostatic, stomachic
阿魏 (Ah-wei)	Asafoetida	Gum-resin	*Ferula assafoetida* (L.) (Umbelliferae)	Vermicide, sedative, antispasmodic, digestive

Chinese Name (Alpha Name)	Common Name	Part Used	Scientific Name (Family Name)	Medical Uses
細辛 (Hsi-hsin)	Asarum	Herb	*Asarum sieboldi* Miq. (Aristochiaceae)	Analgesic, sedative, expectorant
陽起石	Asbestos	Mineral		Stimulant, aphrodisiac
天門冬 (Tien-men-tong)	Asparagus	Root	*Asparagus cochinchinensis* Merr. (Liliaceae)	Diuretic, expectorant
紫菀 (Tzu-wan)	Aster	Root	*Aster tartaricus* L.f. (Compositae)	Antitussive, expectorant

Chinese Name (Alpha Name)	Common Name	Part Used	Scientific Name (Family Name)	Medical Uses
黄耆 (Huang-chi)	Astragalus	Root	*Astragalus hoantchy* Franchet (Leguminosae)	Tonic, diuretic, antipyretic
白朮 (Pai-chu)	Atractylodes (White Atractylodes)	Rhizome	*Atractylodes ovata* DC. A. *macrocephala* Koidz. (Compositae)	Aromatic, tonic, chronic gastroenteritis
蒼朮 (Tsang-chu)	Atractylodes	Rhizome	*Atractylodes ovata* DC. A. *lancea* DC. (Compositae)	Aromatic, tonic, chronic gastroenteritis
橘皮 (Chu-pi)	Aurantium	Fruit rind	*Citrus aurantium* L. (Rutaceae)	Stomachic, digestant, diaphoretic, expectorant, antitussive, antiemetic

Chinese Name (Alpha Name)	Common Name	Part Used	Scientific Name (Family Name)	Medical Uses
薤白 (Hsieh-pai)	Bakeri	Bulbus	*Allium bakeri* Regel, *A. macrostemon* Bge. (Liliaceae)	Smooth the *ch'i*
竹茹 (Chu-ju)	Bamboo	Stem with outside skin removed	*Phyllostachys nigra* Munro (Gramineae)	Refrigerant, antipyretic, antitussive
竹葉 (Chu-yeh)	Bamboo Leaves	Leaves	*Phyllostachys bambusoide* S. et Z. (Gramineae)	Antipyretic
竹瀝 (Chu-li)	Bamboo Sap	Sap	*Phyllostachys nigra* Munro (Gramineae)	Expectorant, antitussive

Chinese Name (Alpha Name)	Common Name	Part Used	Scientific Name (Family Name)	Medical Uses
熊膽 (Hsiung-tan)	Bear Gall	Gall	*Ursus arctos* L. (Ursidae)	Antiphlogistic, antipyretic, analgesic, antispasmodic
射干 (Yeh-kan)	Belamcanda	Rhizome	*Belamcanda chinensis* (L.) DC. (Iridaceae)	Expectorant, antipyretic, stomachic, purgative
冬瓜子 (Tung-kua-tzu)	Benincasa	Seed	*Benincasa hispida* Cogn. *B. cerifera* Savi. (Cucurbitaceae)	Diuretic
柏子仁 (Po-tzu-jen)	Biota	Seed	*Biota orientalis* (L.) Endl. (Cupressaceae)	Tonic, sedative, lenitive

Chinese Name (Alpha Name)	Common Name	Part Used	Scientific Name (Family Name)	Medical Uses
益智 (I-chih)	Black Cardamon	Seed	*Elettaria cardamonum* Maton (Zingiberaceae)	Stomachic, tonic in gastralgia, enuresis, spermatorrhea
白及 (Pai-chi)	Bletilla	Rhizome	*Bletilla striata* (Thunb.) Reichb. f. (Orchidaceae)	Nourish the muscle, hemostatic
青皮 (Ching-pi)	Blue Citrus Peel	Fruit rind	*Citrus medica* L. (Rutaceae)	Aromatic, stomachic
冰片 (Ping-pien)	Borneol	Crystal	*Dryobalanops aromatica* Gaertn.; *D. camphora* Colebr. (Dypterocarpaceae)	Antiphlogistic, antispasmodic, sedative, antitussive

Chinese Name (Alpha Name)	Common Name	Part Used	Scientific Name (Family Name)	Medical Uses
牛黄 (Niu-huang)	Bos	Calculus	*Bos taurus* var. *domestica* Gmelin (Bovidae)	Antitoxin, cardiotonic, antipyretic, sedative, diuretic
綠礬	Brass	Mineral	Ferrous sulfate	Analgesic
白芥子 (Pai-chieh-tzu)	Brassica	Seed	*Brassica alba* L. (Cruciferae)	Emetic
楮實子 (Chu-shih-tzu)	Broussonetia	Fruit	*Broussonetia papyrifera* Vent. (Moraceae)	Stimulant, diuretic, ophthalmic

Chinese Name (Alpha Name)	Common Name	Part Used	Scientific Name (Family Name)	Medical Uses
鴉膽子 (Ya-tan-tzu)	Brucea	Seeds	*Brucea javanica* Merr. (Simarubaceae)	Anthelmintic
密蒙花 (Mi-meng-hua)	Buddleia	Flower	*Buddleia officinalis* **Max. (Loganiaceae)**	Ophthalmic in nyctalopia, asthen-opia, cataract
蒲黄 (Pu-huang)	Bulrush	Pollen	*Typha angustata* Bory et. Chaub.; *T. latifolia* L. (Typhaceae)	Hemostatic, diuretic, **astringent, desiccant,** vulnerary
柴胡 (Chai-hu)	Bupleurum	Root	*Bupleurum chinense* DC. *B. falcatum* L. (Umbelliferae)	Antipyretic, infunctional amenorrhea

Chinese Name (Alpha Name)	Common Name	Part Used	Scientific Name (Family Name)	Medical Uses
血竭 (Hsieh-chieh)	Calamus Gum	Resinous secretion	*Calamus draco* Willdenow (*Daemonorops draco* Blume) (Palmae)	Astringent, hemostatic, analgesic
寒水石 (Han-sui-shih)	Calcite	Mineral	$CaCO_3$	Antipyretic
火麻仁 (Huo-ma-jen)	Cannabis Seed	Seed	*Cannabis sativa* L. (Cannabinaceae)	Tonic, emollient
茵陳 (Yin-chen)	Capillaris	Herb	*Artemisia capillaris* Thunb. (Compositae)	Diuretic, antipyretic in icterus

Chinese Name (Alpha Name)	Common Name	Part Used	Scientific Name (Family Name)	Medical Uses
砂仁 (Sa-jen)	Cardamon	Fruit	*Amomum xanthioides* Wall.; *Hedychium coronarium* Koen. (Zingiberaceae)	Aromatic, stomachic, carminative
紅花 (Hung-hua)	Carthamus	Flower	*Carthamus tinctorius* L. (Compositae)	Uterine astringent in dysmenorrhea
決明子 (Chueh-ming-tzu)	Cassia Seed	Seed	*Cassia tora* L. (Leguminosae)	Various eye and hepatic disorders
兒茶 (Erh-cha)	Catechu	Resin	*Acacia catechu* (L.) Willd. (Leguminosae)	Astringent, refrigerant, antidiarrheic

Chinese Name (Alpha Name)	Common Name	Part Used	Scientific Name (Family Name)	Medical Uses
青葙子 (Ching-hsiang-tzu)	Celosia	Seed	*Celosia argentea* L. (Amaranthaceae)	Ophthalmic
秦艽 (Chin-chiu)	Chin-Chiu	Root	*Gentiana macrophylla* Pall. (Gentianaceae)	Antipyretic, diuretic, exsiccant
青礞石 (Ching-meng-shih)	Chlorite	Mineral	Micaceous earth (A silicate of iron, magnesium, and aluminum)	Expectorant, digestive, antispasmodic
菊花 (Chu-hua)	Chrysanthemum	Flower	*Chrysanthemum morifolium; C. indicum* (Compositae)	Sedative, refrigerant in headache, influenza

Chinese Name (Alpha Name)	Common Name	Part Used	Scientific Name (Family Name)	Medical Uses
蟬蛻 (Chan-shui)	Cicada	Exuviae	*Cryptotympana atrata* Fabr. (Cicadidae)	Antipyretic
升麻 (Sheng-ma)	Cimicifuga	Root	*Cimicifuga dahurica* Maxim. *C. foetida* L. (Ranunculaceae)	Antipyretic, sedative, analgesic
朱砂 (Chu-sha)	Cinnabar	Mineral	Red mercuric sulfide	Antispasmodic, sedative in nervous tachycardia, infantile convulsions
桂枝 (Kuei-chih)	Cinnamon	Ramulus	*Cinnamomum cassia* Blume (Lauraceae)	Aromatic, stomachic

Chinese Name (Alpha Name)	Common Name	Part Used	Scientific Name (Family Name)	Medical Uses
桂皮 (Kuei-pi)	Cinnamon	Bark	*Cinnamomum cassia* Blume (Lauraceae)	Astringent, tonic, analgesic, stimulant
鹿茸 (Lu-jung)	Cervus	Velvet horn	*Cervus nippon* Temminck; *C. elaphus* L. (Cervidae)	Tonic, stimulant
鹿角膠 (Lu-chiao-chiao)	Cervus Colloid	Cervus horn processed by long cooking	*Cervus nippon* Temminck; (Cervidae)	Nutrient, nourish the liver and kidney
鹿角 (Lu-chiao)	Cervus Horn **(Deer Horn)**	Horn	*Cervus nippon* Temminck; *C. elaphus* L. (Cervidae)	Dispel effused blood, improve circulation

Chinese Name (Alpha Name)	Common Name	Part Used	Scientific Name (Family Name)	Medical Uses
木瓜 (Mu-kua)	Chaenomeles	Fruit	*Chaenomeles lagenaria* Koidz. (Rosaceae)	Astringent in diarrhea, analgesic in arthralgia, gout, cholera
櫻皮 (Ying-pi)	Cherry Bark	Bark	*Prunus yedoensis* Matsumura (Rosaceae)	Astringent, antitussive
枳殼 (Chih-ko)	Chih-Ko	Ripe fruit	*Citrus kotokan* (Rutaceae)	Excessive sputum, visceral distention, abdominal swelling
枳實 (Chih-shih)	Chih-Shih	Unripe fruit	*Poncirus trifoliata* Rafin. (Rutaceae)	Stomachic for dysentery, tenesmus, antidiarrheic

Chinese Name (Alpha Name)	Common Name	Part Used	Scientific Name (Family Name)	Medical Uses
肉蓯蓉 (Jou-tsung-jung)	Cistanche	Herb	*Cistanche salsa* Benthament et Hooker (Orobanchaceae)	Aphrodisiac, tonic in spermatorrhea, impotence
陳皮 (Chen-pi)	Citrus	Fruit rind	*Citrus nobilis* Lunr. (Rutaceae)	Stomachic, digestant, expectorant, antitussive, anthelmintic
威靈仙 (Wei-ling-hsien)	Clematis	Root	*Clematis chinensis* Osbeck (Ranunculaceae)	Analgesic, rheumatism, antipyretic, diuretic
丁香 **(Ting-hsiang)**	Clove	Flower	*Eugenia caryophyllata* **Thunb. (Myrtaceae)**	Aromatic, carminative, antiemetic, aromatic, stomachic

Chinese Name (Alpha Name)	Common Name	Part Used	Scientific Name (Family Name)	Medical Uses
白豆蔻 (Pai-tou-kou)	Cluster	Fruit	*Amomum cardamomum* L. (Zingiberaceae)	Aromatic, stomachic with antiemetic action
川芎 (Chuan-chiung)	Cnidium	Rhizome	*Cnidium officinale* Makino; *Ligusticum wallichii* Franch. (Umbelliferae)	Sedative, analgesic, emmenagogue
薏苡仁 (I-yi-jen)	Coix	Seed	*Coix lachryma-jobi* L. (Gramineae)	Refrigerant, diuretic, antirheumatic
黄連 (Huang-lien)	Coptis	Root	*Coptis chinensis* Franch; *C. teeta* Wall. (Ranunculaceae)	Bitter stomachic, digestive, antidysenteric

Chinese Name (Alpha Name)	Common Name	Part Used	Scientific Name (Family Name)	Medical Uses
冬蟲夏草 (Tang-chung-hsia-tsao)	Cordyceps	Fungus	*Cordyceps sinensis* (Berk) Sacc. (Hypocreaceae)	Hemostatic, expectorant, aphrodisiac, astringent, sedative
山茱萸 (Shan-chu-yu)	Cornus	Fruit	*Cornus officinalis* Sieb. et Zucc. (Cornaceae)	Astringent, tonic in impotence, spermatorrhea, lumbago, vertigo, night sweats
延胡索 (Yen-hu-suo)	Corydalis	Tuber	*Corydalis ambigua* Cham. et Schiecht. (Papaveraceae)	Sedative, antispasmodic, analgesic in headache, menstrual colic
山楂 (Shan-cha)	Crataegus	Fruit	*Crataegus pinnatifida* Bge. var. *major* N.E. Br. *C. cuneata* Sieb. et Zucc. (Rosaceae)	Digestant, antidiarrheic

Chinese Name (Alpha Name)	Common Name	Part Used	Scientific Name (Family Name)	Medical Uses
巴豆 (Pa-tou)	Croton	Seed	*Croton tiglium* L. (Euphorbiaceae)	Violent purgative in lead colic
鬱金 (Yu-chin)	Curcuma	Rhizome	*Curcuma longa* L. (Zingiberaceae)	Aromatic, stomachic, chologogue, hemostatic
菟絲子 (Tu-szu-tzu)	Cuscuta	Seed	*Cuscuta japonica* Choisy (Convolvulaceae)	Tonic in impotence, spermatorrhea, prostatitis, neurasthenia
白前 (Pai-chien)	Cynanchum	Root	*Cynanchum stauntoni* (Dcne.) Hand.-Mazz. (Asclepiadaceae)	Antitussive, expectorant

Chinese Name (Alpha Name)	**Common Name**	**Part Used**	**Scientific Name (Family Name)**	**Medical Uses**
鎖陽 (Suo-yang)	Cynomorium	Stem	*Cynomorium coccineum* L. (Cynomoriaceae)	Tonic, aphrodisiac, spermatorrhea
香附 **(Hsiang-fu)**	Cyperus	Tubercles	*Cyperus rotundus* L. (Cyperaceae)	Aromatic, stomachic, emmenagogue, sedative, analgesic
蒲公英 (Pu-kung-ying)	Dandelion	Herb	*Taraxacum officinale* Weber (Compositae)	Stomachic, chola-gogue, lactagogue
石斛 (Shih-hu)	Dendrobium	Herb	*Dendrobium nobile* Lindl.; *D. sp.* (Orchidaceae)	Secretagogue, salivant, sedative

Chinese Name (Alpha Name)	Common Name	Part Used	Scientific Name (Family Name)	Medical Uses
瞿麥 (Chu-mai)	Dianthus	Herb	*Dianthus superbus* L. *D. chinensis* L. (Caryophyllaceae)	Diuretic, emmenagogue
常山 (Charng-shan)	Dichroa	Root	*Dichroa febrifuga* Lour. (Saxifragaceae)	Antimalarial, antipyretic
鷓鴣菜 (Che-ku-tsai)	Digenea	Herb	*Digenea simplex* Agardh (Rhodomelaceae)	Anthelmintic
山藥 (Shan-yao)	Dioscorea	Root	*Dioscorea batatas* Decne. (Dioscoreaceae)	Nutrient tonic, digestant in chronic enteritis and diarrhea

Chinese Name (Alpha Name)	Common Name	Part Used	Scientific Name (Family Name)	Medical Uses
續斷 (Hsu-tuan)	Dipsacus	Root	*Dipsacus asper* Wall. (Dipsaeaceae)	Tonic, analgesic, hematic
白扁豆 (Pai-pien-tou)	Dolichos	Seed	*Dolichos lablab* L. (Leguminosae)	Astringent, stomachic, digestant, anthelmintic
龍骨 (Lung-ku)	Dragon Bone	Fossilized bone	Fossilized bones of dinosaurs and other reptiles	Sedative, antispasmodic, tranquilizer
地龍 (Ti-lung)	Earthworm	Worm	*Allolobophora caliginosa* Trapezoides; *Pheretima asiatica* Michaelsen (Megascolecidae)	Antipyretic, bronchodilator, hypotensor

Chinese Name (Alpha Name)	Common Name	Part Used	Scientific Name (Family Name)	Medical Uses
香薷 (Hsiang-ju)	Elsholtzia	Entire herb	*Elsholtzia cristata* Willd. (Labiatae)	Stomachic, carminative, diuretic
麻黃	Ephedra	(see *ma-huang*)		
淫羊藿 (Yin-yang-huo)	Epimedium	Herb	*Epimedium macranthum* Moore et Decne. (Berberidaceae)	Aphrodisiac
枇杷葉 (Pi-pa-yeh)	Eriobotrya	Leaves	*Eriobotrya japonica* Lindl. (Rosaceae)	Antitussive, expectorant

Chinese Name (Alpha Name)	Common Name	Part Used	Scientific Name (Family Name)	Medical Uses
杜仲 (Tu-chung)	Eucommia	Bark	*Eucommia ulmoides* Oliv. (Eucommiaceae)	Tonic, hypotensor with sedative and analgesic effects
大戟 (Ta-chi)	Euphorbia	Root	*Euphorbia pekinensis* Rupr. (Euphorbiaceae)	Purgative, diuretic
䗪蟲 (Che-chung)	Eupolyphaga	Worm body	*Eupolyphaga sinensis* W. (Corydiidae)	Expel effused blood, treat bruises
芡實 (Chien-shih)	Euryale	Seed	*Euryale ferox* Salisb. (Nymphaceae)	Tonic and astringent in spermatorrhea, analgesic in neuralgia, arthralgia

Chinese Name (Alpha Name)	Common Name	Part Used	Scientific Name (Family Name)	Medical Uses
吳茱萸 (Wu-chu-yu)	Evodia	Fruit	*Evodia rutaecarpa* Bentham (Rutaceae)	Stomachic, carminative, stimulant, uterotonic
茴香 (Hui-hsiang)	Fennel	Fruit	*Foeniculum vulgare* Mill. (Umbelliferae)	Carminative, stomachic, stimulant
黃蠟 (Huang-la)	Flava Wax	Wax	*Apis chinensis* (Apidae)	Internal hemostatic, astringent
紫石英 (Tzu-shih-ying)	Fluorite	Mineral	CaF_2	Tranquilizer

Chinese Name (Alpha Name)	Common Name	Part Used	Scientific Name (Family Name)	Medical Uses
連翹 (Lien-chiao)	Forsythia	Fruit	*Forsythia suspensa* Vahl (Oleaceae)	Antipyretic, antiphlogistic
白鮮皮 (Pai-hsien-pi)	Fraxinella	Peel	*Dictamnus dasycarpus* Turcz. (Rutaceae)	Antipyretic
秦皮 (Chin-pi)	Fraxinus	Bark	*Fraxinus rhynchophylla* Hance (Oleaceae)	Astringent, stomachic
伏龍肝 (Fu-lung-kan)	Fu-Lung-Kan	Earth	The Hardened Earth found on the interior bottom of wood-burning kitchen stoves after several years of use	Sedative, antidiarrheic

Chinese Name (Alpha Name)	Common Name	Part Used	Scientific Name (Family Name)	Medical Uses
高良薑 (Kao-liang-chiang)	Galanga	Rhizome	*Alpinia officinarum* Hance (Zingiberaceae)	Stomachic in dyspepsia, gastralgia, chronic enteritis
鈎藤 (Tiao-teng)	Gambir (Uncaria)	Spines	*Uncaria rhynchophylla* Miq. (Rubiaceae)	Sedative, antispasmodic in infantile nervous disorders
急性子 (Chi-hsing-tzu)	Garden Balsam	Seed	*Impatiens balsamina* L. (Balsaminaceae)	Expel effused blood, expectorant
梔子 (Chih-tzu)	Gardenia	Fruit	*Gardenia florida* L. *G. jasminoides* Ellis (Rubiaceae)	Antipyretic, hemostatic, antiphlogistic in jaundice

Chinese Name (Alpha Name)	Common Name	Part Used	Scientific Name (Family Name)	Medical Uses
天麻 (Tien-ma)	Gastrodia	Root	*Gastrodia elata* Blume (Orchidaceae)	Tonic in vertigo, headache, myoneuralgia, rheumatism
阿膠 (Ah-chiao)	Gelatin	Skin	*Equus asinus* L. (Equidae)	Hemostatic
接骨草 (Chieh-ku-tsao)	Gendarussa	Herb	*Gendarussa vulgaris* Nees (Acanthaceae)	Antirheumatic drug for bonesetting
芫花 (Yuan-hua)	Genkwa	Flower	*Daphne genkwa* Sieb. et Zucc. (Thymelaeaceae)	Diuretic, stomachic, antitussive

Chinese Name (Alpha Name)	Common Name	Part Used	Scientific Name (Family Name)	Medical Uses
龍膽 (Lung-tan)	Gentiana	Root	*Gentiana scabra* Bunge (Gentianaceae)	Stomachic
生薑 (Sheng-chiang)	Ginger	Rhizome	*Zingiber officinale* Rosc. (Zingiberaceae)	Stomachic, stimulant, antiemetic
乾薑 (Kan-chiang)	Ginger, dried	Rhizome	*Zingiber officinale* Rosc. (Zingiberaceae)	Stomachic, stimulant, antiemetic
白果 (Pai-kuo)	Ginkgo	Seed	*Ginkgo biloba* L. (Ginkgoaceae)	Astringent, sedative, antitussive in asthma

Chinese Name (Alpha Name)	Common Name	Part Used	Scientific Name (Family Name)	Medical Uses
人参 (Jen-sheng)	Ginseng	Root	*Panax ginseng* C.A. Meyer (Araliaceae)	Tonic, stimulant, aphrodisiac, indicated in neurasthenia, dys-pepsia, palpitation, impotence, asthma
皂角 (Tsao-chiao)	Gleditsia	Fruit	*Gleditsia sinensis* Lam. (Leguminosae)	Stimulant, expectorant
皂刺 (Tsao-chih)	Gleditsia Spine	Stem spine	*Gleditsia sinensis* Lam.(Leguminosae)	Stimulant, expectorant
北沙参 (Pei-sha-sheng)	Glehnia	Root	*Glehnia littoralis* Fr. Schm. (Umbelliferae)	Expectorant, antitussive

Chinese Name (Alpha Name)	Common Name	Part Used	Scientific Name (Family Name)	Medical Uses
石膏 (Shih-kao)	Gypsum (Gyps)	Mineral	gypsum, native calcium sulfate, alabaster, selenite, satinite, terra alba	Sedative, antipyretic, antiphlogistic
代赭石 (Tai-che-shih)	Haematite	Mineral	native brown iron oxide, Fe_2O_3, and clay	Hematonic, anti-emetic, astringent, hemostatic
石決明 (Shih-chueh-ming)	Haliotis (Sea-ear)	Shell	*Haliotis diversicolor* Reeve; *H. gigantea discus* Reeve; *H.ovina* Gmelin (Haliotidae)	Sedative, alterative, hypotensor
茯苓 (Fu-ling)	Hoelen	Fungus	*Poria cocos* Wolf. (Polyporaceae)	Diuretic, sedative, treatment of oli-guresis, insomnia

Chinese Name (Alpha Name)	Common Name	Part Used	Scientific Name (Family Name)	Medical Uses
蟦螬 (Chi-tsao)	Holotrichia	Worm body	*Holotrichia sauteri* Moser; *H. diomphallia* Bates; *Trematodes tenebrioides* Pallas (Scarabaeidae)	Expel extravasated blood, ophthalmic
何首烏 (Ho-sou-wu)	Ho-Sou-Wu	Root	*Polygonum multiflorum* Thunb. (Polygonaceae)	Tonic, hematogenic
魚腥草 (Yu-hsing-tsao)	Houttuynia	Herb	*Houttuynia cordata* Thunb. (Saururaceae)	Diuretic, urinary antiseptic
血餘炭 **(Hsieh-yu-tan)**	Human Hair	Hair	*Homo sapiens* (L.) (Human hair calcined and powdered) (Hominidae)	Astringent, hemostatic

Chinese Name (Alpha Name)	Common Name	Part Used	Scientific Name (Family Name)	Medical Uses
青黛 (Ching-tai)	Indigo	Pigment	*Indigofera tinctoria* L. (Leguminosae) *Polygonum tinctorium* (Polygonaceae)	Antiphlogistic, anticode, antipyretic
旋覆花 (Suan-fu-hua)	Inula	Flower	*Inula japonica* Thunb.; *I. britannica* L. (Compositae)	Expectorant, stomachic
大棗 (Ta-tsao)	Jujube (Zizyphus)	Fruit	*Zizyphus sativa* Gaertn. (Rhamnaceae)	Nutrient tonic, sedative in insomnia, neurasthenia,
燈心草 (Teng-hsin-tsao)	Juncus	Pith	*Juncus communis* Mey.; *J. decipiens* Nakai (Juncaceae)	Diuretic, antiphlogistic

Chinese Name (Alpha Name)	Common Name	Part Used	Scientific Name (Family Name)	Medical Uses
柿蒂 (Shih-ti)	Kaki	Calyx	*Diospyros kaki* L. F. (Ebenaceae)	Lower *ch'i*, treat hiccoughs
甘遂 (Kan-sui)	Kan-Sui	Root	*Euphorbia kansui* Liou (Euphorbiaceae)	Diuretic, expectorant
赤石脂 (Chih-shih-chih)	Kaolin	Mineral	Essentially hydrated aluminum silicate	Astringent
藁本 (Kao-pen)	Kao-Pen	Root	*Ligusticum sinense* Oliv.; *Nothosmyrnium japonicum* Miq. (Umbelliferae)	Sedative, analgesic

Chinese Name (Alpha Name)	Common Name	Part Used	Scientific Name (Family Name)	Medical Uses
昆布 (Kun-pu)	Laminaria	Herb	*Laminaria japonica* Aresch. (Laminariaceae)	Alterative
馬勃 (Ma-po)	Lasiosphaera	Fungus	*Lasiosphaera nipponica* (Kawam.) Y. Kobayashi et Y. Asahina **(Lycoperdaceae)**	Astringent, antiphlogistic, antitussive, hemostatic
益母草 (I-mu-tsao)	Leonurus	Herb	*Leonurus sibiricus* L. (Labiatae)	Emmenagogue, diuretic, vasodilator
葶藶子 (Ting-li-tzu)	Lepidium	Seed	*Lepidium apetalum* Willd.; *Draba nemorosa* L. (Cruciferae)	Expectorant, diuretic

Chinese Name (Alpha Name)	Common Name	Part Used	Scientific Name (Family Name)	Medical Uses
甘草 (Kan-tsao)	Licorice	Root	*Glycyrrhiza uralensis* Fisch. (Leguminosae)	Demulcent, expectorant, emollient in peptic ulcer
百合 (Pai-ho)	Lily	Bulb	*Lilium japonicum* Thunb. (Liliaceae)	Nutrient, antitussive, expectorant
烏藥 (Wu-yao)	Lindera	Root	*Lindera strychnifolia* Vill. (Lauraceae)	Aromatic, stomachic
紫草 (紫根) (Tzu-tsao)	Lithospermum	Root	*Lithospermum erythrorrhizon* Sieb. et Zucc. (Boraginaceae)	Antipyretic, depuratant in viriola

Chinese Name (Alpha Name)	Common Name	Part Used	Scientific Name (Family Name)	Medical Uses
龍眼肉 (Lung-yen-jou)	Longan	Aril	*Euphoria longana* (Lour.) Steud. *(Nephelium longana* Lam.) (Sapindaceae)	Nutrient tonic in neurasthenia, insomnia
金銀花 (Chin-yin-hua)	Lonicera	Flowers	*Lonicera japonica* Thunb. (Caprifoliaceae)	Diuretic, refrigerant, antiphlogistic, antidiarrheic
淡竹葉 (Tan-chu-yeh)	Lophatherum	Herb	*Lophatherum gracile* Brongniart (Gramineae)	Diuretic, refrigerant
桑寄生 (Sang-chi-sheng)	Loranthus	Entire plant	*Loranthus parasiticus* (L.) Merr. (Loranthaceae)	Tonic, antiphlogistic, hypotensor

Chinese Name (Alpha Name)	Common Name	Part Used	Scientific Name (Family Name)	Medical Uses
蓮房 (Lien-fang)	Lotus Peduncle	Peduncle	*Nelumbo nucifera* Gaertn. (Nymphaceae)	Hemostatic
蓮子 (Lien-tzu)	Lotus Seed	Seed	*Nelumbo nucifera* Gaertn. (Nymphaceae)	Tonic, diarrhea
蓮鬚 (Lien-hsu)	Lotus Stamens	Stamens	*Nelumbo nucifera* Gaertn. (Nymphaceae)	Astringent
水燈香 (Shui-teng-hsiang)	Ludwigia	Root and stem	*Ludwigia octovalvis* (Jacq.) Raven (Onagraceae)	Antipyretic, diuretic

Chinese Name (Alpha Name)	Common Name	Part Used	Scientific Name (Family Name)	Medical Uses
地骨皮 (Ti-ku-pi)	Lycium Bark	Root epidermis	*Lycium chinense* Mill. (Solanaceae)	Antipyretic, anti-tussive in pulmonary tuberculosis
枸杞子 (Kou-chi-tzu)	Lycium Fruit	Fruit	*Lycium chinense* Mill. (Solanaceae)	Nutrient tonic in diabetes, mellitus, pulmonary tuberculosis
海金沙 (Hai-chin-sha)	Lygodium	Spore	*Lygodium japonicum* (Thunb.) Sw. **(Schizaeaceae)**	Antiphlogistic, diuretic, dysuria
茜草 (Chien-tsao)	Madder	Root	*Rubia cordifolia* L. (Rubiaceae)	Emmenagogue, hemostatic

Chinese Name (Alpha Name)	Common Name	Part Used	Scientific Name (Family Name)	Medical Uses
厚朴 (Hou-pu)	Magnolia Bark	Bark	*Magnolia officinalis* Reh. et Wils. (Magnoliaceae)	Antispasmodic, stomachic, antiseptic
辛夷 (Hsin-i)	Magnolia Flower	Flower	*Magnolia liliflora* Desr. (Magnoliaceae)	Tonic, analgesic in sinusitis, rhinitis, coryza, headache, vertigo
麻黄 (Ma-huang)	Ma-Huang	Stem	*Ephedra sinica* Stapf (Ephedraceae)	Bronchial asthma, hay fever, trachitis
麥芽 (Mai-ya)	Malt	Fruit	*Hordeum vulgare* L. (Gramineae)	Stomachic, digestant

Chinese Name (Alpha Name)	Common Name	Part Used	Scientific Name (Family Name)	Medical Uses
膠飴 (Chiao-i)	Maltose	Fruit	*Oryza sativa* L. *Triticum aestivum* L. (Gramineae)	Tonic
桑螵蛸 (Sang-piao-chiao)	Mantis	Chrysalis	*Paratenodera sinensis* de Saussure; *Mantis religiosa* L. (Mantidae)	Nourish the kidney, tonic in impotence, spermatorrhea, enuresis
乳香 (Ju-hsiang)	Mastic	Resin	*Pistacia lentiscus* L. (Anacardiaceae) *Boswellia glabra* (Burseraceae)	Analgesic, sedative, antitussive, expectorant
蜂蜜 (Feng-mi)	Mel (honey)	Honey	*Apis cerana* Fabr. *A. chinensis* (Apidae)	Astringent, demulcent, anti-diarrheic, analgesic

Chinese Name (Alpha Name)	Common Name	Part Used	Scientific Name (Family Name)	Medical Uses
甜瓜蒂 (Tien-kua-ti)	Melo Pedicel	Pedicel	*Cucumis melo* L. (Cucurbitaceae)	Expectorant, emetic
薄荷 (Po-ho)	Mentha	Leaves	*Mentha arvensis* L. var. *piperascens* Malinv. (Labiatae)	Stomachic, carminative, stimulant, diaphoretic
鉛丹 (Chien-tan)	Minium	Mineral	Red lead oxide, Pb_3O_4	Externally as disinfectant, antiphlogistic in conjuctivitis, cuts, and burns
芒硝 (Mang-hsiao)	Mirabilitum	Mineral	Mirabilitum	Cathartic, diuretic

Chinese Name (Alpha Name)	Common Name	Part Used	Scientific Name (Family Name)	Medical Uses
桑白皮 (Sang-pai-pi)	Morus	Root epidermis	*Morus alba* L. (Moraceae)	Antitussive, expectorant in asthma, bronchitis, cough
桑枝 (Sang-chih)	Morus Branch	Branch	*Morus alba* L. (Moraceae)	Antirheumatic, diuretic
桑椹 (Sang-chen)	Morus Fruit	Fruit	*Morus alba* L. (Moraceae)	Tonic
桑葉 (Sang-yeh)	Morus Leaves (Mulberry Leaves)	Leaves	*Morus alba* L. (Moraceae)	Influenza, headache

Chinese Name (Alpha Name)	Common Name	Part Used	Scientific Name (Family Name)	Medical Uses
木鼈子 (Mu-pieh-tzu)	Momordica	Seed	*Momordica cochinchinensis* Spreng. (Cucurbitaceae)	Dispel swelling, detoxifier
牡丹皮 (Mu-tan-pi)	Moutan	Root bark	*Paeonia moutan* Sims (Ranunculaceae)	Antipyretic, emmenagogue, for infections of the digestive tract
烏梅 (Wu-mei)	Mume	Unripe fruit	*Prunus mume* Sieb. et Zucc. (Rosaceae)	Stomachic, antipyretic, astringent
麝香 (She-hsiang)	Musk	Secretion	*Moschus moschiferus* L. (Dried secretion from preputial follicles of the musk deer) (Cervidae)	Cardiotonic, stimulant

Chinese Name (Alpha Name)	Common Name	Part Used	Scientific Name (Family Name)	Medical Uses
肉豆蔻 (Jou-tou-kou)	Myristica	Fruit	*Myristica fragrans* Houtt (Myristicaceae)	Dispel swelling, stimulant
没藥 (Mo-yao)	Myrrh	Resin	*Commiphora myrrha* Engler (Burseraceae)	Exsiccant, stomachic, antispasmodic
川骨 (Chuan-ku)	Nuphar	Root	*Nuphar japonica* DC. (Nymphaceae)	Hemostatic, astringent
五倍子 (Wu-pei-tzu)	Nutgalls	Galls	*Rhus chinensis* Miller (*R. semialata* Murray) (Anacardiaceae)	Astringent, styptic

Chinese Name (Alpha Name)	Common Name	Part Used	Scientific Name (Family Name)	Medical Uses
麥門冬 (Mai-men-tong)	Ophiopogon	Root	*Ophiopogon japonicus* *Liriope spicata* Lour. (Liliaceae)	Antitussive, expectorant, emollient, antiscrofulous
橘紅 (Chu-hung)	Orange Peel	Exocarp	*Citrus reticulata* Blanco (Rutaceae)	Expectorant
粳米 (Keng-mi)	Oryza	Seed	*Oryza sativa* L. (Gramineae)	Tonic, stomachic
牡蠣 (Mu-li)	Oyster Shell	Shell	*Ostrea gigas* Thunb.; *O. talienwhanensis* Crosse; *O. rivularis* Gould (Ostreidae)	In hyperchlorlydria

Chinese Name (Alpha Name)	Common Name	Part Used	Scientific Name (Family Name)	Medical Uses
芍藥 **(Shao-yao)**	Paeonia **(Peony)**	Root	*Paeonia lactiflora* Pall. *P. albiflora* Pall. (Ranunculaceae)	Gastric disorders, intestinal antiseptic, expectorant, emmenagogue
白薇 (Pai-wei)	Pai-Wei	Root	*Cynanchum atratum* Bge. (Asclepiadaceae)	Diuretic, antipyretic
紫蘇葉 (Tzu-su-yeh)	Perilla	Leaves	*Perilla frutescens* Britt. (Labiatae)	Antitussive, stomachic, antiseptic
紫蘇子 (Tzu-su-tzu)	**Perilla Fruit**	**Fruit**	*Perilla frutescens* Britt. (Labiatae)	Antitussive, stomachic, antiseptic

Chinese Name (Alpha Name)	Common Name	Part Used	Scientific Name (Family Name)	Medical Uses
桃仁 (Tao-jen)	Persica	Seed	*Prunus persica* (L.) Batsch (Rosaceae)	Antitussive, sedative in hypertension
前胡 (Chien-hu)	Peucedanum	Root	*Peucedanum dercursivum* Max. (Umbelliferae)	Analgesic, antipyretic, expectorant
牽牛子 (Chien-niu-tzu)	Pharbitis	Seed	*Ipomoea hederacea* Jacq. *(Pharbitis hederacea* Choisy) (Convolvulaceae)	Cathartic, diuretic, anthelmintic
赤小豆 (Chih-hsiao-tou)	Phaseolus	Seed	*Phaseolus calcaratus* Roxb. (Leguminosae)	Diuretic, dispel effused blood, antipyretic, detoxifier

Chinese Name (Alpha Name)	Common Name	Part Used	Scientific Name (Family Name)	Medical Uses
黃蘗 (Huang-po)	Phellodendron	Bark	*Phellodendron amurense* Rupr. (Rutaceae)	Stomachic, antiseptic, externally as antiphlogistic in skin diseases
蘆根 (Lu-ken)	Phragmites	Rhizome	*Phragmites communis* Trin. (Gramineae)	Stomachic, antiemetic, antipyretic
葦莖 (Wei-ching)	Phragmites stem	Stem	*Phragmites communis* Trin. (Gramineae)	Stomachic, antiemetic, antipyretic
商陸 (Shang-lu)	Phytolacca (Pokeberry)	Root	*Phytolacca esculenta* Vanh.; *P. acinosa* Roxb. (Phytolaccaceae)	Diuretic

Chinese Name (Alpha Name)	Common Name	Part Used	Scientific Name (Family Name)	Medical Uses
半夏 (Pan-hsia)	Pinellia	Tuber	*Pinellia tuberifera* Breitenbach (Araceae)	Antiemetic, sedative, antitussive in nausea, pharyngalgia, hiccoughs, chronic gastritis
蓽茇 (Pi-pa)	Piper (Long Pepper)	Fruit	*Piper longum* L. (Piperaceae)	Aromatic, stomachic, analgesic
紫河車 (Tzu-ho-che)	Placenta	Placenta	*Homo sapiens* L. (Hominidae)	Impotence, neurasthenia, infecundity
車前子 (Che-chien-tzu)	Plantago	Seed	*Plantago asiatica* L. (Plantaginaceae)	Diuretic, expectorant

Chinese Name (Alpha Name)	**Common Name**	**Part Used**	**Scientific Name (Family Name)**	**Medical Uses**
桔梗 **(Chieh-keng)**	Platycodon	Root	*Platycodon grandiflorum* A. DC. (Campanulaceae)	Expectorant
遠志 (Yuan-chih)	Polygala	Root	*Polygala tenuifolia* Willd. (Polygalaceae)	Expectorant, cardiotonic, renal tonic
玉竹 (Yu-chu)	Polygonatum	Rhizome	*Polygonatum canaliculatum; P. officinale* All. (Liliaceae)	Tonic
萹蓄 (Pien-hsu)	Polygonum	Herb	*Polygonum aviculare* L. (Polygonaceae)	Diuretic, anthelmintic, antidiarrheic, antiphlogistic

Chinese Name (Alpha Name)	Common Name	Part Used	Scientific Name (Family Name)	Medical Uses
豬苓 (Chu-ling)	Polyporus	Fungus	*Grifola umbellata* Pilat. (Polyporaceae)	Arrests local hemorrhages
夏枯草 (Hsia-ku-tsao)	Prunella	Inflorescence	*Prunella vulgaris* L. (Labiatae)	Alterative, antipyretic, diuretic in scrofula, gout
三七 (San-chi)	Pseudoginseng	Root	*Panax pseudoginseng* Wall. (Araliaceae)	Hemostatic, analgesic
補骨脂 (Pu-ku-chih)	Psoralea	Seed	*Psoralea corylifolia* L. (Leguminosae)	Tonic, stimulant

Chinese Name (Alpha Name)	Common Name	Part Used	Scientific Name (Family Name)	Medical Uses
葛根 (Ko-ken)	Pueraria	Root	*Pueraria thunbergiana* Benth.; *P. pseudo-hirsuta* Tang et Wang (Leguminosae)	Antipyretic, refrigerant
葛花 (Ko-hua)	Pueraria Flower	Flower	*Pueraria thunbergiana* Benth.; *P. pseudo-hirsuta* Tang et Wang (Leguminosae)	Antipyretic, refrigerant
羌活 (Chiang-huo)	Chianghuo	Rhizome	*Notopterygium sp.* (Umbelliferae)	Diaphoretic
使君子 (Shih-chun-tzu)	Quisqualis	Fruit	*Quisqualis indica* L. (Combretaceae)	Vermifuge

Chinese Name (Alpha Name)	Common Name	Part Used	Scientific Name (Family Name)	Medical Uses
萊菔子 (Lai-fu-tzu)	Raphanus	Seed	*Raphanus sativus* L. (Cruciferae)	Stomachic, expectorant
地黃 (Ti-huang)	Rehmannia	Rhizome	*Rehmannia glutinosa* Libosch. (Scrophulariaceae)	Cardiotonic, diuretic, hemostatic in diabetes mellitus
大黃 (Ta-huang)	Rhubarb	Rhizome	*Rheum palmatum* L. *R. officinale* Baill. (Polygonaceae)	Stomachic in gastric catarrh and diarrhea
金櫻子 (Chin-ying-tzu)	Rosa Fruit	Fruit	*Rosa laevigata* Michx. (Rosaceae)	Carminative, astringent tonic

Chinese Name (Alpha Name)	Common Name	Part Used	Scientific Name (Family Name)	Medical Uses
覆盆子 (Fu-pen-tzu)	Rubus	Fruit	*Rubus chingii* Hu; *R. coreanus* Miq. (Rosaceae)	Astringent
番紅花 (Fan-hung-hua)	Saffron	Stigm	*Crocus sativus* L. (Iridaceae)	Improve the circulation, antipyretic
丹參 (Tan-sheng)	Salvia Root	Root	*Salvia miltiorrhiza* Bunge (Labiatae)	Female tonic in amenorrhea, metrorrhagia, gastralgia, mastitis
檀香 (Tan-hsiang)	Santalum	Wood	*Santalum album* L. (Santalaceae)	Aromatic stomachic, carminative, analgesic in nervous gastralgia

Chinese Name (Alpha Name)	Common Name	Part Used	Scientific Name (Family Name)	Medical Uses
蘇木 (Su-mu)	Sappan-Wood	Wood	*Caesalpinia sappan* L. (Leguminosae)	Hemostatic, astringent
海藻 (Hai-tsao)	Sargassum	Herb	*Sargassum fusiforme* (Harv.) Setch. (Sargassaceae)	Diuretic, used for iodine deficiencies
木香 **(Mu-hsiang)**	Saussurea	Root	*Saussurea lappa* Clarke (Compositae)	Treatment of asthma, stomachic
五味子 (Wu-wei-tzu)	Schizandra	Fruit	*Schizandra chinensis* Baillon (Magnoliaceae)	Tonic, stimulant, antitussive

Chinese Name (Alpha Name)	Common Name	Part Used	Scientific Name (Family Name)	Medical Uses
荊芥 (Ching-chieh)	Schizonepeta	Whole Herb	*Schizonepeta tenuifolia* Briq. (Labiatae)	Diaphoretic, antipyretic
三稜 (San-leng)	Scirpus	Rhizome	*Scirpus martimus* L. (Cyperaceae) ***Sparganium ramosum*** Huds. (Sparganiaceae)	Emmenagogue, analgesic, laxative
全蠍 (Chuan-hsieh)	Scorpion	Worm body	*Buthus martensi* Karsch (Buthidae)	Antispasmodic, nerve tonic
玄參 (元參) **(Hsuan-sheng)**	Scrophularia	Root	*Scrophularia ningpoensis* Hemsley (Scrophulariaceae)	Cardiotonic, antipyretic, antiphlogistic

Chinese Name (Alpha Name)	Common Name	Part Used	Scientific Name (Family Name)	Medical Uses
黄芩 (Huang-chin)	Scute	Root	*Scutellaria baicalensis* Georgi (Labiatae)	Stomachic, antipyretic, expectorant
小薊 (Hsiao-chi)	Segetum	Herb	*Cirsium segetum* Bge. (Compositae)	Dispel effused blood, cool the blood, hemostatic
海螵蛸 **(Hai-piao-chiao)**	Sepia **(Cuttlebone)**	Sepsium	*Sepia esculenta* Hoyle (Sepiidae)	**Strengthen the body,** increase circulation, hemostatic
胡麻仁 (Hu-ma-tzu)	Sesame	Seed	*Sesamum indicum* L. (Pedaliaceae) *Linum usitatissimum* L. (Linaceae)	As lenitive in scybalous constipation; as nutrient tonic in degenerative neuritis or neuroparalysis

Chinese Name (Alpha Name)	Common Name	Part Used	Scientific Name (Family Name)	Medical Uses
粟米 (Su-mi)	Setaria	Seed	*Setaria italica* L. Beauv. (Gramineae)	Nourish the spleen, digestive, stomachic
豨薟草 (Hsi-chien-tsao)	Siegesbeckia	Herb	*Siegesbeckia pubescens* Mak.; *S. orientalis* L. (Compositae)	Analgesic, antirheumatic
防風 (Fang-feng)	Siler	Root	*Siler divaricatum* Benth. et Hook.; *Ledebouriella seseloides* Wolff. (Umbelliferae)	Antipyretic, analgesic
殭蠶 (Chiang-tsan)	Silk-worm	Worm	*Bombyx mori* L. (Bombycidae)	Sedative, analgesic, expectorant

Chinese Name (Alpha Name)	Common Name	Part Used	Scientific Name (Family Name)	Medical Uses
土茯苓 (Tu-fu-ling)	Smilax	Root	*Smilax china* L. *S. glabra* Roxb. (Liliaceae)	Alterative, diuretic in syphilis, gout, skin disorders, rheumatism
淡豆豉 (Tan-tou-shih)	Soja	Preparation	*Glycine max* (L.) Merr. (Leguminosae)	Antipyretic
苦參 (Ku-sheng)	Sophora	Root	*Sophora flavescens* Ait. (Leguminosae)	Bitter stomachic, astringent in dysentery, enterorrhagia
八角茴香 (Pa-chiao-hui-shiang)	Star Anise	Fruit	*Illicium verum* Hook. (Magnoliaceae)	Stomachic, stimulant

Chinese Name (Alpha Name)	Common Name	Part Used	Scientific Name (Family Name)	Medical Uses
百部 (Pai-pu)	Stemona	Root	*Stemona sessilifolia* (Miq.) Franch et Savat.; *S. tuberosa* Lour. (Stemonaceae)	Antitussive, pediculicide
防己 (Fang-chi)	Stephania	Root	*Stephania* tetrandra S. Moore (Menispermaceae)	Antipyretic, diuretic, analgesic, arthritis, lumbago, myalgia
硫黃 (Liu-huang)	Sulfur	Mineral	The innate sulfur after a preliminary processing	Vermicide, laxative
蝱蟲 (Mang-chung)	Tabanus (Gadfly)	Worm	*Tabanus mandarinus* Schi.; *T. bovinui* (Tabanidae)	Emmenagogue

Chinese Name (Alpha Name)	Common Name	Part Used	Scientific Name (Family Name)	Medical Uses
滑石 (Hua-shih)	Talc	Mineral	Native Hydrous Magnesium Silicate, $3MgO \cdot 4SiO_2 \cdot H_2O$	Antiphlogistic, hemostatic, diuretic
當歸 (Tang-kuei)	Tang-Kuei	Root	*Angelica sinensis* Diels (Umbelliferae)	Emmenagogue, sedative, analgesic
黨參 (Tang-sheng)	Tang-Sheng	Root	*Codonopsis tangshen* Oliver (Campanulaceae)	Tonic in anemia, chronic enteritis, weak stomach tone
細茶 (Hsi-cha)	Tea	Leaves	*Thea sinensis* L. *(Camellia sinensis* Kuntze) (Theaceae)	Cardiotonic, central nerve stimulant, diuretic, intestinal astringent

Chinese Name (Alpha Name)	Common Name	Part Used	Scientific Name (Family Name)	Medical Uses
訶子 (Ho-tzu)	Terminalia	Fruit	*Terminalia chebula* Retz. (Combretaceae)	Astringent, hemostatic, antidiarrheic, antitussive
通草 (Tung-tsao)	Tetrapanax	Pith	*Tetrapanax papyrifera* (Hook) K. Koch (Araliaceae)	Diuretic, galactagogue
敗醬 (Pai-chiang)	Thlaspi	Herb	*Thlaspi arvense* L. (Cruciferae); *Patrinia scabiosaefolia* Link. (Valerianaceae)	Antipyretic, detoxifier, improve circulation, dispel pus, expectorant, diaphoretic
蟾蜍 (Tsan-chu)	Toad	Body	*Bufo bufo gargrizans* Cantor; *Bufo melanostictus* Schneider (Bufonidae)	Expel moisture and fever, dispel swelling, analgesic, detoxifier

Chinese Name (Alpha Name)	Common Name	Part Used	Scientific Name (Family Name)	Medical Uses
蟾酥 (Tsan-shu)	Toad Secretion	Secretion	*Bufo bufo gargarizans* Cantor; *Bufo melanostictus* Schneider (Bufonidae)	Detoxifier, analgesic, tonic, diuretic
萆薢 (Pi-hsieh)	Tokoro	Root	*Dioscorea sativa* L. *D. tokoro* Makino **(Dioscoreaceae)**	Diuretic
鼈甲 (Pieh-chia)	Tortoise Shell	Carapace	*Amyda sinensis* (Trionychidae)	Antipyretic, tonic
菱角 (Ling-chueh)	Trapa	Fruit	*Trapa natans* L. (Trapaceae)	Tonic, antipyretic

Chinese Name (Alpha Name)	Common Name	Part Used	Scientific Name (Family Name)	Medical Uses
蒺藜 (Chi-li)	Tribulus	Fruit	*Tribulus terrestris* L. (Zygophyllaceae)	Tonic, astringent
栝樓 (天花粉) (Kua-lou)	Trichosanthes Root	Root	*Trichosanthes kirilowii* Max. (Cucurbitaceae)	Antipyretic
栝樓子 (Kua-lou-tzu)	Trichosanthes Seed	Seed	*Trichosanthes kirilowii* Max. (Cucurbitaceae)	Antitussive, expectorant, emollient for skin swellings
草果 (Tsao-ko)	Tsao-Ko	Fruit	*Amomum tsao-ko* Crevost et Lem. (Zingiberaceae)	Digestive, expectorant

Chinese Name (Alpha Name)	Common Name	Part Used	Scientific Name (Family Name)	Medical Uses
草豆蔻 (Tsao-tou-kou)	Tsao-Tou-Kou	Seed	*Alpinia katsumadai* Hay. (Zingiberaceae)	Stomachic
獨活 (Tu-huo)	Tuhuo	Root	*Angelica laxiflora* Diels *A. grosseserrata* Maxim. (Umbelliferae)	Antispasmodic, analgesic, diaphoretic, diuretic
薑黃 (Chiang-huang)	Turmeric	Rhizome	*Curcuma aromatica* Salisb. (Zingiberaceae)	Dispel effused blood, emmenagogue, analgesic
槲寄生 (Hu-chi-seng)	Viscum	Entire plant	*Viscum album* L. (Loranthaceae)	Hypotensor, lactagogue, antiphlogistic

Chinese Name (Alpha Name)	Common Name	Part Used	Scientific Name (Family Name)	Medical Uses
蔓荊子 (Mian-ching-tzu)	Vitex	Fruit	*Vitex rotundifolia* L. *V. trifolia* L. (Verbenaceae)	Sedative, analgesic
浮小麥 (Fu-hsiao-mai)	Wheat	Fruit	*Triticum aestivum* L. (Gramineae)	Sedative, antipyretic
紫藤瘤 (Tzu-teng-liu)	Wisteria	Gall	*Wisteria florabunda* D.C. (Leguminosae)	Stomachic, antiphlogistic
烏頭 (Wu-tou)	Wu-Tou	Root	*Aconite carmichaeli* Debx. (Ranunculaceae)	Antispasmodic, sedative, analgesic

Chinese Name (Alpha Name)	Common Name	Part Used	Scientific Name (Family Name)	Medical Uses
蒼耳子 (Tsang-erh-tzu)	Xanthium	Fruit	*Xanthium strumarium* L. (Compositae)	Antipyretic, antispasmodic, diaphoretic
川椒 (Chuan-chiao)	Zanthoxylum	Fruit	*Zanthoxylum piperitum* DC.; *Z. simulans* Hance (Rutaceae)	Stimulant, tonic, stomachic, carminative, diuretic
椒目 (Chiao-mu)	Zanthoxylum Seed	Seed	*Zanthoxylum simulans* Hance (Rutaceae)	Diuretic, edema and swelling
酸棗仁 (Suan-tsao-jen)	Zizyphus (Jujuba)	Seed	*Zizyphus jujube* Mill. *Z. sativa* var. *spinosa* (Rhamnaceae)	Nutrient tonic, sedative, insomnia, neurasthenia